YOU SAY I HAVE WHAT??

"Living With Cancer And A Rare Disease, Amyloidosis"

Dr. Dez

YOU SAY I HAVE WHAT??
"Living With Cancer And A Rare Disease, Amyloidosis"

Dr. Dez

All rights reserved. No part of this book may be reproduced or transmitted in any form or by any means without written permission from the author.

Unless otherwise noted, all Biblical versions are from
The New King James Version

U.S. Copyright © 2023 1-12209111621

Published by © 2023 DSC Publishers, Inc.
All rights reserved.

ISBN: 979-8-218-13234-7

Printed in the U.S.A.

DEDICATION

This book is dedicated to my family:

Darryl J. Holliday, my husband, has supported me and loved me unconditionally since the beginning. He is my biggest cheerleader, motivating and encouraging me never to give up.

To my children, Arnay Marshall, Calvin Marshall, and Malicia Johnson, and godchildren, Tyrone, Kelly Pronty, and Jennifer Gerrell, who uplifted and provided their unwavering support.

They help to make my life complete.
They are the reason for my why.

ACKNOWLEDGEMENTS

First, I want to acknowledge God, my Lord, and Savior. Without Him, I would not be here. He has given me the inspiration and strength to write this book. Next, I want to acknowledge my family and friends who prayed for me during this challenging time. So many days, they reached out to provide encouragement and support. I am forever grateful to them.

FOREWORD

I had the pleasure of reading one of Dr. Dez's initial writings years ago. What captured my attention was the unextinguishable fire she exemplified, chronicling the Word of God. Subsequently, I surmised that for someone who possesses such power and anointing, Dr. Dez has undoubtedly been a woman in the presence of her Lord and Savior, Jesus Christ.

It is an honor to write the foreword.

However, I believe "fireword" would better exemplify the anointing placed on her life, to the first of many books to be written by this powerful woman of God.

Dr. Desiree-Love-Holliday has written this book as though her life was set ablaze by God and used her life and health experiences as true-to-life testimonies.

This book is a testimony to assist other believers in pressing forward and defying the odds of overcoming disease, sickness, and life-threatening issues. Her boldness and proactive involvement in helping others who encounter various illnesses are highlighted, as well as her encounter of coming to a place of conditioned healthiness.

The simplicity and openness of her journey are captivating and encouraging to anyone who will peruse the pages of this publication with an openness to gain a wealth of experience and encouragement.

This writing sends a profound message that you can do all things through Christ, who strengthens you. Trusting God is another strong message she features in this book. Her testimonies are where you will genuinely find her faith activated, alive, and aligned with God.

Dr. Dez underscores the importance of family, friends, and faith-filled intercessors. These support groups were instrumental in nurturing her back to mental, physical, and spiritual well-being.

Although this book may have been dark at times, the light in Dr. Dez prevailed through her resilience, perseverance, and faith in God. This assurance demonstrated in this book

Also, I would be remiss if I failed to mention those in the medical profession whom God used and has continued to use to replenish, renew, restore, and bring my friend, Dr. Dez, to the place of wholeness and wellness. Each word will enlighten your soul, dispelling any hopes of darkness's attempt to hold you bound in what you feel or have been made to think that there is no other alternative but to accept your dark condition.

Reap the many blessings presented to you in this Holy Spirit-filled book.

Be open.
Be encouraged.
Be blessed.
Be healed.

These four areas of encouragement are expressed in this dynamic book.

Jehovah-Rophe,
Annie Brown, Pastor
Praying House Ministries, Inc.
Wives Who Pray, Founder
Hasten to His Throne, Founder
A Ready Builder Enterprise
Certified Professional Life Coach

CONTENTS

Introduction 9

Chapter 1: The Beginning 19

Chapter 2: Amyloidosis 39

Chapter 3: My New Normal 62

Chapter 4: Stem Cell 71

Chapter 5: Emotional Whirlpool 92

Chapter 6: Gaining Emotional Support 104

Chapter 7: Spiritual Prescription 113

Chapter 8: Taking Control 139

Chapter 9: Future Recommendations 151

Conclusion 165

Healing Scriptures 172

Thank You 176

Bibliography 177

Contact 180

INTRODUCTION

I can't change the direction of the wind,
but I can adjust my sails always to reach my destination.
Anonymous

Bombshell! Unbelievable! I was in for the shock of my life. I did not see this coming by a long shot. I felt like I was blindsided.

Something is approaching, coming in for a landing that I can't see. I have no control over it. An unforeseen life-changing moment that I can't even put into words. My emotions are all over the place.

I was sitting in the doctor's office, waiting for the test results. The anticipation was killing me, and just waiting for the news. Ten minutes seemed like an hour. Tick toc, tick toc, tick toc. Finally, the doctor came into the room. The wait was over. The doctor started to talk, but I could not hear clearly. My mind went into a whirlwind. Everything was blah, blah, blah. Was the doctor talking to me? Was there someone else in the room beside me? There must be someone else in the room other than me. Not me, definitely not me. Oh yes, the doctor was talking to me. It was like a bell going off in my ear. Dang! Dang! Dang! Wake up! The doctor was talking to me. I can't believe it. I can't fathom what was coming out of the doctor's mouth. The doctor's lips moved in that split second, but I could not comprehend.

Suddenly, the sounds of the doctor's voice seemed muffled. It was a complete blur. The doctor was probably wondering whether she could hear the words coming out of my mouth. I am not saying anything. I am motionless. Then the tears started to stream down my cheeks at the words that came out of the doctor's mouth.

My life as I knew it suddenly stopped and changed in an instant forever. I went to sleep one way and woke up another way. One day I was healthy, and the next day my world changed. This was a nightmare. Let me go back to sleep and wake up again, hoping for a different outcome. WOW! This can't be true. I never believed that something like this could ever happen to me. I never imagined that I would be experiencing a life-changing moment that would transform my life indefinitely. As a matter of fact, for the rest of my life.

There are things in our life where we experience a life-altering event. I thought to myself, not like this. I thought I could handle almost anything that came my way. I had been through a lot in my life, or so I thought. I had to remind myself that I am a SURVIVOR and that I could do this. You have no choice. You have to handle this like a warrior.

Most of the time, the life-changing events we think about are a new job, promotion, marriage, divorce, the birth of a baby, death, moving to a different state or city, relationships (boyfriend, girlfriend), and family dynamics. These are just some of the junctures in our life that might last for a few seconds, a few minutes, a few hours, a few days, maybe weeks, years, or a lifetime. My thought process was that you have at least some control, if not all, over every situation, and you can make adjustments when necessary. Most of the time, we do. Right?

After all, it is our life, and we are responsible for handling what happens to us, good or bad. It is up to us to adjust to the change and decide what actions to take. How we deal with change is supposed to be our personal choice and responsibility. Hopefully, these life-altering events will be handled efficiently, and one can move forward. But eventually, it all concludes no matter how they alter the circumstances.

So, life happens, and what happens can sometimes be called change. Because we live in this world, things can happen expected or unexpected. We don't like the unexpected, but it happens. The unexpected took place in my life. It shook my world to the core. I was totally shaken. Can I get a break, God? No! Not this! Why me? I go to church. I am faithful. I minister to others. I love God. I can't imagine this happening to me.

What did I do wrong for this to happen to me? I had to snap back to my senses and think realistically. Bad things happen to good people. It is not God's will for me to be sick. If that is the case, why would He heal people in the bible and continue to do so today? Sickness is not of God. I did not expect this to happen at this time in my life. I don't know why, but I didn't. After all, I am basically healthy. So, I thought. This was the last thing that was on my radar. I felt out of control. As the commercial says, **I HAVE FALLEN, AND I CAN'T GET UP! HELP! HELP!**

Change is the one constant in a person's life. When I think about change, there is always a factor of control over the outcome. After all, that is what I learned. You hear about change, speak about change, read about change, but nothing could prepare me for this moment. I know that change can come from various directions and is dealt with differently. Sometimes change comes from the left field, and you can't see it coming. That's me. I was thrown a curveball. It just happened, and I have to deal with it. I had to move from a passive state of mind of observing how things unfold to taking immediate action in my life.

Change is not always easy. Sometimes change is inevitable. We cannot prevent change. Change is what makes the world go round. It is how one reacts to the change that matters. Life doesn't always turn out the way we want it to. Dealing with the unknown can be scary. I was unsure what to expect and began anticipating everything, good or bad. I had to accept and believe I could handle what I had no control over. Most importantly, not only accept what I cannot change but to be able to adjust. My choice is whether to meet the change with grace and acceptance or with protest and resistance.

SERENITY PRAYER

God grant me the serenity

to accept the things I cannot change;

courage to change the things I can;

and wisdom to know the difference.

Living one day at a time;

Enjoying one moment at a time;

Accepting hardships as the pathway to peace;

Taking, as He did, this sinful world

As it is, not as I would have it;

Trusting that He will make all things right

If I surrender to His Will;

So that I may be reasonably happy in this life

And supremely happy with Him

Forever and ever in the next.

It is in these times of unforeseen change that we are truly challenged. I always say that if you live long enough, things will happen that will throw us for a loop. Sometimes we are met with resistance, downpours, and obstacles that don't seem to stop. At times, all three seem to occur at the same time. People say that if it's not one thing, it's another. You conquer one thing, and then another happens, and then another happens, wondering if it will ever stop.

Because I believe there is life and death in the power of the tongue. I choose to speak the opposite of what I see, feel, and hear. I must admit it gets difficult always to say the right thing, and I know I am not the only one who feels that way sometimes, if we are truly honest with ourselves.

While this abrupt life-altering situation interrupted the usual flow of my daily life and disrupted my normal functioning, it afforded me the opportunity and the challenge to re-evaluate my life and alter my way of living. I call it My New Normal. According to Brenner (2011), when we have accepted and mastered the concept of change, it is easier to alter our lives accordingly with the knowledge and trust that we are being carried in its flow.

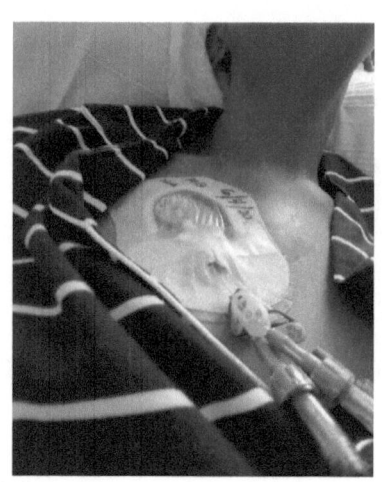 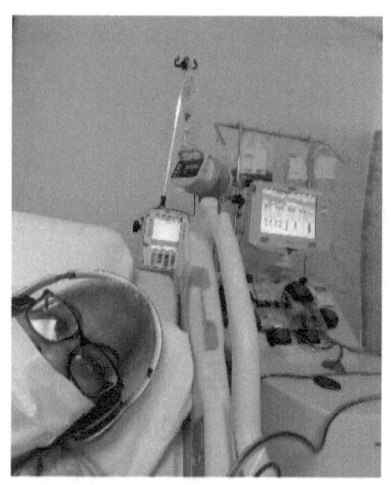
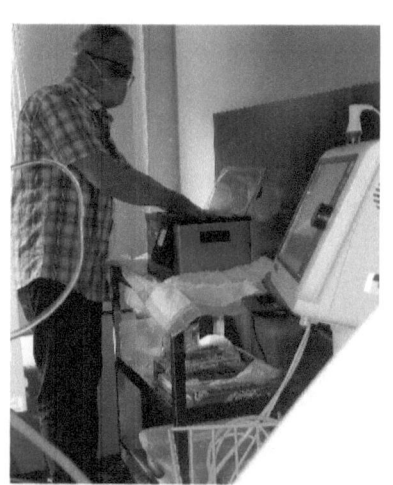 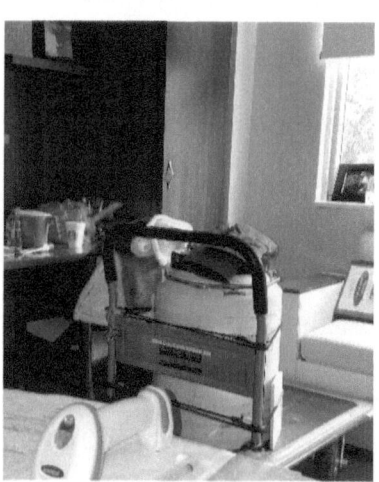

Chapter 1

THE BEGINNING

"But there's a beginning in the end, you know? It's true that you can't reclaim what you had, but you can lock it up behind you. Start fresh."
Alexandra Bracken,
The Darkest Minds

Reflecting on my illness, I believe it all started sometime in 2017. My husband thinks my illness escalated after a road trip we took to see our son in Louisiana in September 2017. He believes the trip stressed my body since we did not rest much before returning home. It was a long road trip. At the time, my husband and I were working and returned immediately to work upon returning from visiting my son. I have to agree that my illness seemed to escalate upon our return. Immediately, I got sick and had to go to the emergency room a week or two later. I had breathing problems, so I went to the ER. The doctors took all types of tests and found nothing. I stayed overnight in the hospital for observation and went home the next day, still not feeling well. From that point, everything started to go downhill.

Before my diagnosis, I had several emergency room visits that resulted in six observation stays and one admission to the hospital for shortness of breath and chest pain. During this timeframe, it included several visits to various doctors (pulmonologist, gastroenterologist, three cardiologists, and primary care) and numerous medical tests that all returned negative. I took so many medical tests that I should have lit up like a light bulb. Every place I went, I should have automatically lit up any room. I felt like I had an automatic radiant glow from all the radiation my body took from the multiple tests I took in a short period of time.

At one point, my doctor thought I was suffering from psychological issues such as depression when everything else physically failed. Depression was causing me to be sick. It appeared to be psychosomatic. Really! Since the doctor had known me for several years and my medical history, it was a surprise that the doctor would think I was suffering from some type of mental health issue. The doctor was starting to get just as perplexed as I was feeling.

Of course, I told the doctor I was not depressed about anything, which was the truth. I was not having any problems at home and/or at my job. Everything was good. I did not feel well and did not know why. I believed my family and friends, including my husband, thought it was psychological. The doctor was baffled but did not give up. During this same time period, I lost a lot of weight. I was fatigued, losing weight without effort, had shortness of breath, and felt totally sick.

I told the doctor something was wrong. Thank God! My doctor would not give up on me. She felt something was wrong but didn't know why. One of the doctor's statements was," Over the years, I have attempted to get you to lose weight with very little success. Now you are losing weight without any effort. Something is definitely wrong, but we have not solved the problem yet."

Mystery

Mystery #1 that went unnoticed and misdiagnosed was that I started getting dark pigmentation underneath my eyes that would not go away and was not hereditary. It was not getting better, only getting worse. Getting darker and darker, it seemed, by the day. I asked my cousin if she noticed this underneath our grandmother's eyes. She stated that our grandmother did not have this problem.

Further, my cousin indicated that she did not have a problem with darkness underneath the eyes, nor did any other relative in the family.

Next, I spoke to my pulmonologist, and the doctor felt it was allergies. Yes, I have allergies, but that was not the cause of the darkness underneath and around my eyes. Nonetheless, allergies can cause some darkness, but it was eventually discovered that this was not the case with me. In addition, the doctor started treating me for asthma, which contributed to my shortness of breath. The doctor was trying every combination of medication, and after several visits to the office, I seemed only to feel better for a short while and then get sick again.

Mystery #2 was chest pain and shortness of breath. As mentioned, I went to the hospital several times, including hospital stays. Medical tests were taken at the hospital and on an outpatient basis, including EKGs, blood tests, echocardiograms, CT chest pulmonary embolism exam, chest x-rays, stress test, nuclear stress test, and a 24-hour heart monitor. Each time the test returned negative or showed no sign indicating that I should be experiencing this level of difficulty with my heart. I visited two different cardiologists, and the problem was not resolved. As a result, another doctor's appointment was scheduled for a follow-up. The problems remained. My primary care physician continued to have other medical tests completed. The mystery continued.

Mystery #3 Excessive unexplained weight loss. Losing weight? Who does not want to lose weight? I do not know many ladies who do not want to lose weight effortlessly, even if it is one pound. So, when I started losing weight, I thought this was great. I went down a dress size, so I figured this was fantastic! Then I kept losing more weight over a short period of time. I was not on a diet and did nothing special to lose weight. Every time I went back to the doctor, I lost a bit more weight. To say the least, she was not highly ecstatic about the continued weight loss. The doctor started questioning me about the weight loss. More medical tests were ordered and doctor office visits. When I kept losing weight without effort, I knew deep inside that something was wrong. My family and friends stated that I did not look well. In fact, I started to look sickly. The weight loss continued more quickly. I lost a total of fifty-seven pounds in less than a year without being on a diet.

Mystery #4 Office visit with my primary doctor. This time my husband accompanied me to my doctor's visit. He thought I was keeping information away from him. I tried to comfort him by telling him everything that I knew he knew about my health. However, he still thought I was keeping secrets and insisted on coming with me. He was extremely worried but did not want to show it.

As my doctor came into the room, she gave him the same information I had already given him. Since we both have the same doctor, she was very comfortable providing information. Besides, HIPPA was signed by both of us, permitting the doctor to release medical information. We had a no-hold-bars conversation. She even asked him if there was a problem at home. WOW! Who would ever think a primary doctor would think of asking such a question to my spouse? I guess she figured she would get to the bottom of this problem.

Medical instinct kicked in, and she asked me to stick out my tongue. Lo and behold, I had a huge tongue. She turned to my husband and said, "Did you notice that your wife's tongue was so large?" He looked amazed and stated, "I had never seen her tongue that large."

The mystery now started to unravel. My doctor indicated I had to go for a biopsy and referred me to a doctor who would perform the biopsy. Since I was taking so many tests, I did not think to ask the doctor why I needed a biopsy. It was just another test to try to solve the mystery. Later my doctor told me that she did not want to tell me her suspicions until she got confirmation. She suspected that I had Amyloidosis.

There is an Amyloidosis Center in Israel; she had seen many patients with Amyloidosis while studying medicine. I thank God for Dr. Rotem Amir. I attribute her steadfastness to helping to save my life.

It was not any of the doctor's fault that Amyloidosis was not the initial diagnosis. Many doctors do not think about this disease and/or misdiagnose the disease. This happens to many people who are diagnosed with Amyloidosis. The only way to get confirmation is through a biopsy.

Amyloidosis mimics many medical conditions such as shortness of breath (asthma, heart), kidney problems, gastrointestinal, weight loss and neuropathy, etc. Many people who suffer from Amyloidosis can go undiagnosed for years. Unfortunately, some people are diagnosed later than sooner. Some people die due to irreversible organ damage while waiting for a diagnosis. The disease is very rare. I am one of the blessed who received a so-called early diagnosis.

Mystery Starts To Unravel

While walking through this unknown journey, I was required to complete my annual mammogram and bilateral ultrasound. In September 2018, I completed my exam. The doctor returned and indicated that a mass had appeared on my breast. I needed to come back and have a biopsy. Since I had a breast biopsy completed several years ago, I did not think there would be any problem.

At that time, a clip was placed to monitor a specific area in the breast. There weren't any differences every year that I returned, so I wondered why this year should be any different. Therefore, I took my slow time to schedule the biopsy. After all, I was not worried. This issue does not have anything to do with me being sick.

My co-workers were surprised that I did not immediately schedule the biopsy. Finally, in December 2018, I scheduled the biopsy.

Another ultrasound was conducted, and the doctor decided to wait for those results prior to performing another biopsy. The doctor mentioned that a biopsy would not be completed at the time because they wanted to see if there was any mass growth. Return in six months, the biopsy would be completed if needed, and another ultrasound would be conducted to determine if a biopsy was necessary. I did not hesitate to adhere to the doctor's instructions this time. So, in June 2018, I scheduled the biopsy. An ultrasound was taken, and the mass had grown. The breast biopsy was completed. I waited for the results, which would take two weeks.

Mystery Unraveled

I returned home and told my husband the results would not be back for another two weeks. So now, instead of one-person thinking about the results, we were both somewhat concerned. However, we did not think the breast biopsy was connected to my being sick. So now, the wait started. The clock goes tick tock, tick tock for the next two weeks.

I was still going to see another doctor to have another biopsy, as instructed by my primary doctor. This biopsy was related to my huge tongue. I contacted the doctor to have the biopsy completed in the stomach area, called a fat pad biopsy. An appointment was scheduled. The doctor's office called and indicated that they needed my medical records from the primary doctor's office before I came to the appointment. As a result, I contacted my primary doctor to send the information. I received a call the day before the appointment and was informed that they had received the information and that I could come to the office the next day. Of course, I canceled because I simply did not want to go. I told them I could not come the next day because I could not get time off from work with such short notice. I lied. I did not want to have two biopsies within the same timeframe. I rescheduled the doctor's appointment for a fat pad biopsy a month later.

Eventually, the pad fat biopsy appointment was canceled due to a diagnosis I received from the breast biopsy. It was not necessary.

The wait is over, or so I thought. While at work, on a Friday, I received a call from the primary care physician's office.

I thought I would hear good news. Who wants to hear bad news? I was informed that I had to come into the doctor's office because the test results were back, and the doctor wanted to discuss them with me. When I heard that, I knew automatically that something was wrong. Ninety-nine percent of the time, the doctor never wants to see you unless something is wrong. Now I was officially worried.

Next, I was told the doctor does not work on Friday, so I had to wait until Monday. I was so upset that the doctor's office called me on a Friday and told me the doctor would not be available until Monday the following week. I had to wait an entire weekend before I knew the results. I contacted my husband, and the first thing we thought about was the Big C, cancer. To say the least, our weekend was ruined. All that was on our minds was that I had breast cancer. We did not say much about it to each other, but this was constantly on our minds.

On Monday morning, we went to the doctor's office. We went inside the room with high anticipation. The wait for the doctor seemed like an eternity, almost unbearable. Finally, the doctor entered the room. She spoke in such a soft tone, smiling like she always does, that we thought everything was okay. The doctor stated that you don't have breast cancer. My husband and I sighed with a false sense of relief. In our minds, my husband and I thought great. Good news. But the next thing that came out of the doctor's mouth shook our world. "You do not have breast cancer, but they found amyloid in your breast." What? What? What was the doctor talking about? The doctor stated, "You have Amyloidosis." I have what? At that point, everything seemed to go mumbo jumbo.

I did not hear anything after the word Amyloidosis. I was diagnosed with a disease I could not say and/or understand.

As I already described, the doctor was talking to me, and I could not hear anything. My world stopped. It was like a motion picture. I was in one frame, and the other frames kept moving without me. Then I heard that I was sending you to an oncologist/hematologist. I fell apart. Even though the diagnosis was awful, I was happy to have the diagnosis. Finally, people would stop thinking that I was imagining that I was not feeling well. Nope, I was not going crazy.

The next stop was to the oncologist/hematologist, who attempted to explain the diagnosis again. I could not wrap my head around what the doctor was saying. I was in total shock. The last thing I expected was to hear that I have a rare disease that had no cure called AL Amyloidosis. I had never heard of this. The doctor indicated that he wanted me to have another biopsy completed, called a bone marrow biopsy, to confirm the original diagnosis. I learned it is very unusual to find amyloid in the breast. So now I was to have another biopsy. It was something I did not want to do, but I did not have any other choice. The only way to confirm the diagnosis of the disease was through a biopsy. I had to wait two weeks to complete the biopsy because there were no openings. Then I would wait almost another two weeks to see the oncologist. The wait was agonizing.

While waiting, I was a psychological wreck. This cannot be real. I felt like I had an out-of-body experience. I was walking around but could not comprehend anything. I cried most of the time. I couldn't speak to anyone without crying. My mind was swirling around and around. It was overloaded. I was sitting at work, just going through the motions. I want to scream!

Finally, after four weeks, the wait was over. I went to the doctor's office, and it was confirmed that I had a dreaded disease called AL Amyloidosis. The first question I asked was, "Is this hereditary?" The doctor indicated that my type is AL Amyloidosis, which is not hereditary. Thank God, my children would not get this disease from me. At least, I hope and pray this will never happen to them. Even though the doctor says my children will not get the disease, it remains on my mind because there is a hereditary type. The second question was, "How did I get it?" The doctor could not tell me how I got the illness. It is something that just happened to me. WOW! Really! What did I do to deserve this? The third question was, "How is this treated? Chemotherapy was his response. This was the last thing I thought about ever having to do in this lifetime. The fourth question I asked was this cancer?" No, I was told Amyloidosis is not cancer.

Next, it was determined that I had a form of Multiple Myeloma, a blood cancer. This cannot be real. Multiple Myeloma did not compute for many months later because the oncologist was concentrating on the Amyloidosis. They are both blood disorders and are treated in the same manner. I guess the doctor figured I would have a total meltdown if I connected the dots between Amyloidosis and Multiple Myeloma. The doctor was probably right. There was only so much that I could take.

Many questions followed every time I went to the oncologist in charge of my treatment. In my case, I found out later that if I did not have Multiple Myeloma, I would not have AL Amyloidosis. Not that it makes me feel any better. It does not. They are both incurable diseases.

When I learned about my diagnosis, I started living My New Normal. I went to sleep one day and woke up with a rare disease called AL Amyloidosis and Multiple Myeloma.

I cannot do anything about it except fight it with every fiber of my being. My New Normal is what it is.

Fight The Good Fight Of Faith
1 Timothy 6:12

Chapter 2

AMYLOIDOSIS

I don't expect to live forever, but I intend to hang on as long as possible.

Isaac Asimov

Everyone has heard of Multiple Myeloma, which is blood cancer, but hardly anyone has heard of AL Amyloidosis. When people hear about cancer, the following questions might be asked: "Well, what type of cancer is it?" What happens next?

I was informed that I have Multiple Myelomas. In my case, it is connected with AL Amyloidosis, which is not cancerous. However, they both involve the blood system, a bone marrow disorder. Multiple Myeloma symptoms occur at different levels of progression. Multiple Myeloma is a cancer of the plasma cells. Plasma cells live in our bone marrow.

The bone marrow is where all the blood cells are formed. These plasma cells are part of the immune system and functionally produce antibodies, a type of protein to help deal with infections. These plasma cells grow like any other cell in our bodies. When they grow more than ten percent of all the cells in the bone marrow, the diagnosis is called Multiple Myeloma. Multiple Myeloma is a rare form of cancer, accounting for only zero-point seventy-six percent (1 in 132) of all new cancers in the U.S. (American Cancer Society, 2021).

Only ten percent of people diagnosed with AL Amyloidosis have Multiple Myeloma. Most people who have Multiple Myeloma have the disease located in their bones. I do not have the bone lesions that can be present in people who have been diagnosed with Multiple Myeloma. Thank God mine had not progressed that far. Periodically, doctors conduct bone scans to check for the detection of bone involvement.

For the purpose of this book, I will discuss AL Amyloidosis since it is a rare disease. I get a strange and confused look when I tell people about AL Amyloidosis. What is that? When I was told, I was flabbergasted.

Between the crying, tears, and smiles of relief and victory, every individual diagnosed with AL Amyloidosis lives and distinctively reacts to the disease. Depending upon whom you speak to, you will get a different account of the degree of difficulty in treating the disease, the side effects of chemotherapy, and recovery from organ damage. Every person has a different journey. However, there are many similarities, and one common denominator is that all AL Amyloidosis patients have to do chemotherapy and/or Stem Cell Transplant. Depending upon the type of Amyloidosis, some individuals get an organ transplant.

When patients receive an Amyloidosis diagnosis, they do not know what to do or where to travel. Generally, patients are in total darkness with this rare and serious disease. It's like a softball coming from left field that you do not see. It hits you like a huge rock. The road to complete recovery can be short or long. The doctors have told me that patients are never in complete remission like cancer but can obtain a "complete response." The term that references remission in Amyloidosis is called "a complete response." First, it is called "a complete response" because there is a positive and/or total response to treatment. Secondly, there is another type of remission called a "very good partial response," partial remission. Lastly, no response. Most doctors say remission because most people understand the term more easily.

Unfortunately, some people die from the disease, and some live long and happy lives, living their new normal.

So, you might ask what determines whether a person lives or dies. It depends upon when the individual received their initial diagnosis and how badly the disease damages the organs. The earlier the diagnosis, the better to maximize the healing process from the disease.

Unfortunately, many people are not diagnosed immediately because this disease mirrors many other conditions. Many individuals do not get diagnosed until the disease has advanced. The last thing many doctors think about is Amyloidosis. Numerous doctors do not come across it in their practice, so they do not think about it. In the United States, approximately 4,500 new cases are diagnosed yearly (Amyloidosis Foundation, 2020). Typical Amyloidosis symptoms are shortness of breath, fatigue and weakness, numbness, tingling or pain in the hands or feet, irregular heartbeat, enlarged heart, impaired voice, a rash of small purplish spots or red spots, darkness under the eyes (skin changes), diarrhea and/or constipation, urine changes, unintentional/significant weight loss, abnormally large tongue, swelling of the ankles and legs, difficulty swallowing, carpal tunnel syndrome and dizziness when standing. Symptoms depend on which organs are affected.

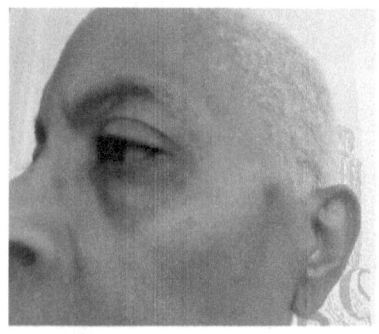
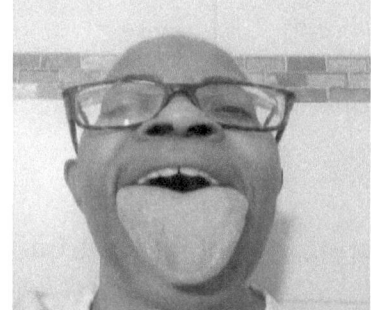

Do you know some of the symptoms of AL Amyloidosis?

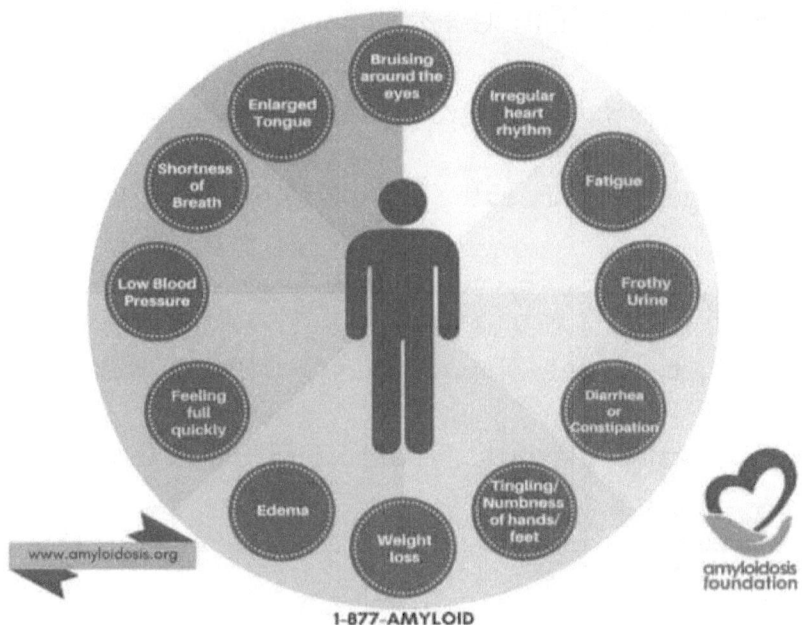

As I mentioned earlier in the book, it was a difficult road prior to being diagnosed with Amyloidosis. On this journey to final diagnosis, an individual's experience is similar to mine prior to obtaining a diagnosis. For many people, there was a minimum of one year or more before a diagnosis of Amyloidosis was obtained which included several doctor office visits, medical tests, and hospital stays. I was diagnosed in a year. My diagnosis was considered early. Go figure?

Once I was officially diagnosed with AL Amyloidosis, I immediately went online to research my diagnosis and learn everything I could about the disease. The doctors do not want you to go online because some information might be outdated, confusing, and/or incorrect. But I went online anyway, against the doctor's advice and knowledge. Nothing could keep me from going online and researching. This can be good or bad. For me, it was a combination of both. At the onset, I was more confused than ever because I was reading information I did not completely understand. Some posts made me feel like I was going to die tomorrow. Prepare for the funeral and tell my family goodbye.

Reading all of the information made me feel overwhelmed. In my mind, I was saying are they talking about me?

No, not me. Not really me! There was medical documentation, terms I had never heard of and did not understand entirely, including others' personal testimonies. I was inundated with information. There was so much to learn and understand. Today, I am still learning and continue to seek answers. It is like entering a new world, one that has never been discovered, and now I am searching for answers, and everything sounds and looks strange. I was definitely afraid of the fact that I had AL Amyloidosis. There were so many underlying symptoms. Who knew? I want to make it clear that it takes specific tests performed to confirm a diagnosis.

Confusion Sets In

I was confused and perplexed. Then it got more confusing because of some of the responses I received. To keep people's anonymity, I did not include the names, just the responses I listed below to demonstrate the wide range of information. For example, I asked, is Amyloidosis cancer or not cancer? The answers went from one end of the spectrum to the next, yes to no, and all in between. Some of the responses may be correct or incorrect. It is all opinions. This is just a small caption of what I received because the responses were numerous. Here goes:

- I'm confused too!
- The first oncologist I went to, the first thing he said to me was, "you've got cancer."
- Not technically cancer since no tumors form
- I would tell people it's a cousin to bone marrow cancer.
- Told not cancer but treated the same way.
- It should be cancer. My husband has been doing chemo for six years now.

- They don't say it's not cancer, but I feel soon they will categorize it as such.

- Doctors told us Amyloidosis is a precancerous form of Multiple Myeloma.

- The disease is similar to multiple myeloma, which is a bone cancer. The two diseases are treated similarly, although the amyloid process is not considered cancer.

- It's an autoimmune disease.

- My husband was diagnosed with blood cancer, which caused amyloidosis.

- This AL Amyloidosis is complicated to understand because many problems and complications arise. For example, one minute, you can feel good and full of energy, then the next, you feel weak and down, etc... it's an unpredictable disease.

- There's primary, secondary, and heredity amyloidosis. Primary amyloidosis is caused by advanced multiple myeloma, a blood cancer.
- They don't know what causes any of the Amyloidosis types. Additionally, you can have Multiple Myeloma, Amyloidosis, or both.
- I hate when people say that at least it's not cancer! My wife has been through hell and still battling!
- So, I call it cancer, but as I said, some of my colleagues don't.

Whew! Mind-boggling. With all that being said. I am no closer to the truth than when I started getting responses from fellow patients. Unfortunately, I could not get a definitive answer. However, I did get some information that attempted to assist me in understanding this complicated disease. My hematologist/oncologist, considered one of the experts in the field, indicated that it is hard to explain to some doctors.

Let's Ask The Professionals

Medical Community states:

AL amyloidosis is related to a type of bone marrow cancer called multiple myeloma. It is treated similarly with chemotherapy drugs and sometimes with stem cell transplantation. However, amyloidosis is not cancer (Cancer.Net Editorial Board, 2016).

Great, this is not cancer. So, what is this Amyloidosis?

There are different types of Amyloidosis which are Primary or Secondary Amyloidosis, AL Amyloidosis, AA Amyloidosis, ATTR Amyloidosis, and Localized Amyloidosis.

All of which are treated differently. I have AL Amyloidosis, a systematic disease. This type of Amyloidosis is not hereditary.

Amyloidosis is a rare disease. The United States classifies a rare disease as affecting less than 200,000 people (National Disorders for Rare Disorders, 2020). Currently, rare diseases affect 3.5% - 5.9% of the worldwide population. Allergies and environmental factors can cause rare diseases, bacterial and/or viral infections, degenerations, and proliferative or genetic diseases. Amyloidosis is a serious condition. If the condition is left untreated, it is progressive and can lead to death.

It is estimated that about 4,000 people develop AL Amyloidosis each year in the United States (Cancer.Net Editorial Board). It usually affects individuals between the ages of 50-80 years of age. However, some cases affect individuals as young as someone in their 20's. Hereditary or Non-Hereditary (ATTR), Cardiac Amyloidosis, and AA amyloidosis are less common than AL amyloidosis.

Most people are diagnosed with AL Amyloidosis. Early diagnosis is imperative for the survival of the individual. The later the diagnosis, the more difficult to treat and recover.

Amyloidosis is a condition that affects various tissues and organs of the body. Because it is rare and unusual, the disease is problematic and difficult to diagnose. The symptoms and severity of amyloidosis can vary between individuals, although some symptoms are more common than others.

Due to significant medical advancements, the outlook of individuals with Amyloidosis has dramatically improved. Presently, there is no cure for Amyloidosis.

However, there can be an extended period of time in which an individual can be symptom-free. As a result, they can live long and healthy lives. Twenty years ago, the life expectancy of patients diagnosed with amyloidosis was only a few months or years. Currently, the survival rate is ten years or more (amyloidosis.org.uk).

AL Amyloidosis

As mentioned, AL Amyloidosis is the most common type of amyloidosis in individuals diagnosed within the United States and other countries. AL Amyloidosis is a systematic disorder. The disease starts in the bone marrow. The bone marrow is located in the center of the bones that produces cells in the system called plasma cells, which make antibodies (immunoglobulins) that assist the body in protecting itself against infection. Plasma cells are located mainly in the bone marrow.

Additionally, bone marrow creates red blood cells, white blood cells, and platelets. After the antibodies have finished their job, the body breaks them down. When the bone marrow cells produce antibodies that cannot be broken down,

Amyloidosis comes into being. The antibodies build up in the blood and eventually get deposited in the tissues as amyloid (misfolded protein deposits). These abnormal proteins, called amyloid, build up and overproduce in the bone marrow called light or heavy chains, interfering with the organ's normal function.

Due to the overproduction of amyloid, it leaves the bone marrow and attaches itself to vital organs in the body. The best way to think of it is like the links of a chain connected that does not come apart. Unfortunately, too many links go to unwanted places, such as the body's organs, nerves, and tissues. Amyloidosis can affect the heart, kidneys, liver, spleen, and nervous system. Amyloid deposits can ultimately impair organs and cause them to stop working if left untreated. AL Amyloidosis does not affect the brain.

Occasionally Amyloidosis can manifest when an individual has certain forms of cancer, such as multiple myeloma, Hodgkin's disease, or familial Mediterranean fever (an intestinal disorder). Additionally, the disease might occur in people with kidney disease who have undergone dialysis for a long time (Cedars Sinai, 2019).

On the other hand, some people do not even have symptoms, which makes the condition more difficult to diagnose. When Amyloidosis is associated with another disease, indicators may be hidden. The underlying disease may be fatal before Amyloidosis is found (Cedars Sinai, 2019). The cause for amyloid to be produced and collected in the tissues is unknown. The risk of amyloidosis is not connected to what an individual eats, lifestyle, or stress.

Diagnosis

Amyloidosis often goes unnoticed because the signs and symptoms can mimic those of more universal diseases. Consequently, early diagnosis can help stop the disease's further progression.

Precise diagnosis is important because treatment varies greatly, depending on your specific condition. Therefore, only your doctor can diagnose the disease.

Amyloidosis cannot be diagnosed only with a simple blood and/or urine test. Diagnostic testing for AL Amyloidosis involves blood tests, urine tests, imaging tests, and biopsies. With a biopsy, the samples are stained with a Red Congo Stain that reacts with the amyloid to determine the diagnosis. If Hereditary Amyloidosis is detected, the physician might conduct genetic testing.

Treatment

Depending upon the type of Amyloidosis and symptoms, the treatment varies. For example, treatment for Hereditary Amyloidosis differs from other types of Amyloidosis. As I mentioned, patients with the same disease experience some of the same symptoms, but the type of treatments and length of treatments vary. Treatment for this disease continues to evolve. It is the hope that one day there will be a cure.

As for myself, I have received chemotherapy, immunotherapy, and a stem cell transplant, with future treatments to be determined. All of this can be overwhelming. Nonetheless, I keep a positive attitude. At times, I do get depressed, but I continue to keep a smiling face, knowing that I am not the only individual who is experiencing a life-threatening condition. Ultimately, God is in total control, the Master planner and future of my life.

You may ask the question why did I choose to receive chemotherapy? Some people felt that I should have gone completely natural treatment. For me, the answer was obvious. I choose chemotherapy to save my life. I did not want to take chemotherapy, but I felt it was my best decision. I had to make a life-and-death decision. I could have worsened my condition if I had waited and decided to go the natural route. Another year my health condition could have looked different to my detriment. I did not want to take the chance. It was not worth it to me. You cannot allow other people's opinions to sway you from what you think is suitable for your life. The choice is yours to make.

I choose not to operate in thoughtlessness or speculation. If you are faced with a life-threatening condition like mine, I advise following the doctors' directions. Yes, you should pray about it and get a spiritual release. I did. If you wait, your condition could get worse.

You should have peace with your decision because the road to go down is not always easy. Anticipating what you heard, saw, and thought about chemotherapy is more harmful than the treatment currently received. Many improvements have been made to how chemotherapy is given to individuals. It is not always a complete nightmare.

People like myself receive chemotherapy and go home the same day after treatment. I am not saying that you might not have side effects. I am just saying that it is better than years ago. Medical science has advanced for the better. Many are living longer and more prosperous lives. The key is early detection and treatment.

I do believe in supernatural healing. However, healing can also come in the form of a doctor. God placed doctors in the earth realm for a reason. Remember, Luke was a physician (Colossians 4:14). If doctors were not needed, they would not be in the earth realm. Just make sure you choose the correct doctor. If you believe and have faith in God, He will get you through it. The Word of God says, *"He will never leave or forsake you. Do not be afraid; do not be discouraged (Deuteronomy 31:8)."*

"Knowledge is of two kinds. We know a subject ourselves or where we can find information on it."

Samuel Johnson

Chapter 3

MY NEW NORMAL

Things that may never go back to normal. You may need to create a new normal. And that's okay.

Johilder.com

Major incidents in our lives can shake our world that prompt us to interact and move within our lives differently. Many events stand out in my life that were significant and molded me as an individual today. Some of these were: I moved out of state, went to college, and graduated, relationships, family, traveled, married, and had children. These events impacted my life in some way, but none compared to what I was about to encounter. I am now in a class of individuals that have experienced a new normal. My life changed forever. One day everything was fine, and the next day everything changed.

You never really think of permanent life-changing circumstances until it happens to you. I believe that sometimes we take life for granted, feeling that nothing major will ever happen until we grow older. It is something that we don't think much about. These days what is old? As days and years pass by, we come to realize that we are not that invincible.

I never really thought about anything medically significant happening in my life. Maybe when I got older, but not now. After all, I still considered myself young at heart and young in age. When I mentioned my age to my Amyloidosis acquaintances, they told me I was a youngster. Compared to them, I was the youngest in the group. Can you believe that? I just laughed. Bear in mind. I thought that I was reasonably healthy, nothing life-threatening. I never believed it would happen to me. Neither did anyone else think that it would happen to them.

My life as I knew it would never be the same again. A shift from the old to the new had taken place. Living with a rare disease and blood cancer is like maneuvering through a winding journey filled with questions, choices, answers, tears, and hopes. I've seen the positive signs of my disease moving in the right direction that get sidetracked by the changes in treatment, the progression of treating the disease, and then only to find out that this was a very long process with possible setbacks.

Previously, normal for me was my daily routine. I went to work and church, visited friends and family, traveled, and thought about starting an exciting new chapter in my life since I had recently completed my doctoral degree. Before, I could happily say I was a wife, mom, friend, minister, and advisor. Now, I am an AL Amyloidosis and Multiple Myeloma patient and survivor, including a wife, mom, friend, minister, and advisor. I went from a so-called everyday life to a life where I had to adjust and conquer.

My new normal is living with AL Amyloidosis/Multiple Myeloma as a constant companion. Currently, how I view myself compared to how others see me has changed. I look and feel different. I am more conscious about how I feel daily. Even when I looked fine, I often did not feel well at some point and time of the day. When people looked at me, I did not seem ill. They thought nothing was wrong with me. I looked like a healthy person with no medical issues. Most of the time, I did not move around like I had an illness. I thank God that I did not look how I felt. This was indeed a blessing.

I thought about the disease in some aspects of my everyday routine. When I was not feeling the side effects of the disease,

I was thinking about my treatment for it or if I would ever be free of it. For example, I couldn't walk past a mirror without being reminded that I have AL Amyloidosis. When I looked in the mirror, I saw the disease's effects. I have darkness around my eyes, the darkness around the sides of my mouth and chin, my tongue is enlarged, and the inside of my mouth becomes easily bruised.

Sometimes I didn't even look in the mirror because I didn't like what I saw. Occasionally, I wore makeup in an attempt to hide what I saw. I wear my glasses more often than I wear my contacts. If I wore my contacts, I wore sunglasses to hide the darkness underneath my eyes. I will only take pictures with my sunglasses and/or my prescription glasses. I do all this to avoid what I see, not necessarily what others see when they look at me. One day, my daughter, whom I had not seen for a while, asked me if I had a suntan which impact what I was thinking about my complexion. At that time, I did not go anywhere that would have caused me to get a suntan. I was not outside enough to get a tan. My complexion was darker due to chemotherapy. Then I questioned my husband, who continues to love me unconditionally. He said hesitantly, yes, you are a little darker. He later told me; he wished my daughter had not said anything because he did not want me to feel bad. So now I just say that I have a chemo tan. This is my new normal.

After the diagnosis of Amyloidosis/Multiple Myeloma, the state of my so-called normal took on a whole new meaning, it turned into going to chemotherapy initially weekly,

bi-weekly, and progressed to monthly, intravenous infusions, and other medical tests. Various needle sticks became routine. Sometimes the nurse and/or the technician could not find my veins. My veins probably got scared from being stuck so many times and decided to disappear. I could almost tell when they would miss the vein by looking at how they attempted to draw the blood and/or get the line for the IV. I could have sworn my veins started to withdraw from fright at one point. I could hear my veins saying, no, I will not cooperate with you today. I'm hiding. You have been here too many times. So, in order to prevent missed sticks, I automatically knew where they could get a good stick and would tell them.

Medication! Medication! I went from six medications I took daily to thirteen when I counted them all. While I was hoping to delete medications, the doctors kept adding medications because my condition contributed to other health conditions. I had to take some medications daily and others on an as-needed basis. This did not include my chemotherapy treatments. Are you overwhelmed yet? I am, so I tried not to think about it. I just did it. My medications represented the ever-present nudge. Don't forget to take your medications.

Remember, you are sick and need these pills to keep you healthy and alive. They supposedly will help to save your life in the long run. Unfortunately, all medications have some type of side effect. Some of which can be unpleasant. Nothing is perfect. I tried to deal with the side effects and/or get a change in medication that usually had another type of side effect. If you thought about it too hard, you would not take any medication. This routine was a constant reminder that this was my new normal.

It was tough to comprehend what I did not fully understand. Further, it was hard to grasp something that had changed my life indefinitely, and I had to accept it. The change that occurred was necessary. I questioned, why did this happen to me? I believe many people ask this question and are afraid to admit it.

Having AL Amyloidosis is like a radio station that I leave on when I leave my home. When I leave, the station is working properly. When I return, the radio station frequency might have shifted, causing me to change it. I have to tune my radio to a new frequency to hear it again. The radio is like having Amyloidosis/Multiple Myeloma. Every day I have to shift to adjust to my new normal, developing a new way of living in a meaningful way. I have to believe the good outweighs the bad. I keep the faith, knowing that God will see me through.

The truth is you don't know what is going to happen tomorrow. Life is a crazy ride, and nothing is guaranteed.

Eminem

Chapter 4

STEM CELL

Sometimes the smallest step in the right direction ends up being the biggest step in your life.

Naeem Callaway

It was a well-thought-out plan. My doctor, Dr. James Hoffman, told me the next step he recommended in my treatment plan was a stem cell transplant. My health condition was better than when I first started treatment. He sent me to the stem cell transplant doctor, Dr. Lazaros Lekakis, who would oversee my stem cell transplant. While I had the stem cell transplant, Dr. Lekakis became the primary physician.

He would become the secondary doctor until the transplant process was completed. Basically, they work as a team. He would be aware of everything that was happening.

I went to my scheduled appointment with Dr. Lekakis. Speaking with the doctor, no problems should occur. Numerous stem cell transplants have been completed without incident. I should be in the hospital for two weeks. Three weeks is the maximum. I am having an autologous stem cell transplant, meaning I am using my stem cells. Before the procedure, healthy stem cells would be taken from my body.

I would not have to worry about incompatibility between donor cells since I was using my cells. However, preliminary tests must be performed to determine whether the stem cell transplant could be conducted safely.

Needless to say, I completed many required tests, such as a dental examination, chest x-ray, blood test, pulmonary function test, echocardiogram, EKG, and an x-ray to examine the bones throughout the body. All tests returned, indicating that I could have the stem cell transplant as planned. On my next visit to the doctor, he reviewed the test results, explained the stem cell transplant process, and ensured that I wanted to proceed.

Once the doctor completed everything he said to pray. Not many doctors acknowledge prayer. I was surprised that he said it. It let me know that he realized there was a power higher than his. Doctors can only go so far; the rest belongs to God. I was in the right place. Next, I had to take medicine to stimulate my stem cells prior to extracting my stem cells. Once this process was completed, I went for the apheresis stem cell collection. The cells are collected, frozen, and stored until used at a later date. All went well without any incidents. Now, I waited for a hospital date which was a week later.

Most importantly, I prayed before going to the hospital and starting the process. Prayer is essential for everything.

Prayer is my connection to God. I believe He hears me when I pray. The Bible says He hears the voice of His children. *"Then you will call on me and come and pray to me, and I will listen to you. You will seek me and find me when you seek me with all your heart. (Jeremiah 29:12-13, NIV)."* I trusted without a doubt that God heard my prayer. First, I believed in God's protection and safety. *Those who go to God Most High for safety will be protected by the Almighty (Psalms 91:1, NCV).*

Secondly, I believed I had received my answer, so I was comfortable proceeding. *"No weapon formed against me shall prosper (Isaiah 54:17, NKJV)."* Overall, I was at complete peace with my decision. As I went into the hospital, I felt a sense of peace and that God was completely covering me.

Going into the hospital was like going into a cocoon or bubble. Nothing could come in and/or go out. The unit was entirely secure. In spiritual terms, I called it Noah's Ark. Once Noah and his household, including the animals, entered the Ark, nothing entered. He was secure and safe during the storm. Noah was under God's complete protection. All of the necessary provisions were inside the ark. Noah followed God's specific instructions and was considered a righteous man. Just like Noah had to follow God's specific instructions, I had to follow the doctor's instructions to avoid harm's way. All the necessary provisions for my recovery and health were inside the hospital.

Once I entered the unit, no one was allowed in or out except the medical staff, dietitian, nutritionist, physical therapist, room service associate, and patient services assistants. Due to the coronavirus pandemic, family members were not allowed to visit. This was the most disheartening part of my admission. Previously, my husband and I discussed delaying the stem cell transplant but decided it was best to proceed. Currently, I am eligible to receive a transplant. The stem cell transplant was initially delayed because of my medical condition and the coronavirus pandemic. If I waited any longer, I might become ineligible due to sudden changes in my medical condition. Anyway, I had already started the process, and why stop now? Delaying the stem cell transplant would cause me to commence the stem cell transplant process from the beginning meaning that I would have to repeat the numerous tests. Many people desired to have a stem cell transplant. However, due to poor medical health, they were ineligible.

My husband dropped me off at the hospital entrance on my arrival date. A transportation worker came to the lobby door, took my suitcases, and placed me in a wheelchair to be escorted upstairs to the stem cell unit. Nonetheless, we smiled and kissed each other before I entered the hospital. I waved goodbye. He watched me as I entered and then left. I did not feel completely alone because I knew God was with me. Nonetheless, I wished my family could visit.

I was placed in a very nice patient room. I called it a mini-suite. Unfortunately, I was the only one who could see it. I placed my family pictures on the windowsill and a plaque that stated, "Be The Kind Of Woman That When Your Feet Hit The Floor Each Morning. The Devil Says, Oh No… She's Up." The staff who entered the room loved my family pictures and the plaque. It gave the room a homier feeling.

The pictures explained why I was doing the stem cell transplant. In the beginning, everything was going well. As explained, I would receive chemotherapy on the first day to kill cancer cells left in the body and make room for new stem cells. On the second day, my stem cells would be reintroduced back into my body. As planned, things went well without a hitch. Next, waiting for my blood level to hit what medical personnel called zero. This I called the waiting period. During this time, I wait for the cells to engraft or take, after which they multiply and make new blood cells. At this point, I was doing fine. No major problems appeared to exist.

Sometimes the unexpected can happen. It happened to me. Surprise! Surprise! A well-made plan that resulted in unforeseen problems. Once my blood level hit zero, the unpredicted happened. I can't remember much after that period. I went into what they call a semi-conscious state.

However, I say I was unconscious because I could not remember anything. Initially, the doctors could not understand and/or determine why this happened.

Next, they called my husband and requested that he come to the hospital, hoping to turn things around, which was against hospital policy because of the coronavirus pandemic. God's favor was on his side. The doctors were very concerned. My husband came to the hospital for three days straight. He stated that I responded to some things. I would say hey repeatedly and slowly sing with him Victory Is Mine, I Told Satan Get Thee Behind. None of this can I recall and still don't remember.

He called my relatives, placing the phone next to my ear and/or FaceTime having them try to talk to me and pray for me. I responded slightly but mostly remained silent. Again, all of which I do not remember. He called everyone that he could think of to pray for me. After three days, he could not return any longer because the doctors felt it would be a health risk to the other unit's patients and me because of the coronavirus pandemic.

If he stayed, he would have to remain at the hospital overnight until discharge which could be a few days later. After three days, when my husband left the hospital, there was no major change in my condition. Periodically, he called the hospital to get an update.

I was given numerous blood tests, CT scans of the abdomen and pelvis, and other tests, including MRI and CT scans of the brain, to determine if I had suffered a brain injury. My husband thought I had a stroke because my face looked droopy.

All of the test results came back negative. After my husband left the hospital, unbeknownst to anyone, a psychiatrist decided to give me a low dose of Haldol since there was no significant change in my condition. My son had called the hospital several times and was always informed that I was sleeping.

Finally, my son became concerned and contacted my husband. The same night my husband contacted the hospital to inquire about my medical condition as he usually did and found out that I had been given Haldol. My husband knew that I could not give authorization, and he did not give permission and/or have knowledge of me receiving such a potent medication. Haldol is a very powerful antipsychotic medication. It treats schizophrenia, psychosis, and severe behavioral problems in children. I do not have a history of psychiatric problems.

To my husband's knowledge, the primary doctor providing oversight of my medical condition was supposed to take me off all medications to clear out my system. The primary doctor thought this could be a solution to resolve my medical problem. My husband inquired about the medication with friends who knew the drug, indicating that I should not receive this medication. The possible side effects were not good and could have bad outcomes.

Further, I never had any psychiatric issues to anyone's knowledge of me. Immediately, my husband contacted the hospital and informed the nurse not to give any further medication until he spoke to the doctor. When the doctor returned to my room the next day, he told the doctor that I had no psychiatric issues and had never had any in my life.

He has been with me for over twenty years and would know. My husband started suggesting different psychiatric lower-grade medications from working with children for many years. The doctor told my husband he was trying to be an at-home pharmacist. Thank God, my husband was looking out for his wife, who could not do for herself. It is blessed to have a husband looking out for your welfare. We are always there for each other.

Without his intervention, I probably would have continued to receive the medication, which would increase my problems and had long-lasting psychological effects. Upon discussion, the medication was immediately stopped. The primary doctor informed my husband that he was unaware that a fellow doctor had recommended and administered the medication.

Eventually, it was determined by the primary doctor that I went into a state of delirium, an alteration of consciousness. He had seen it before, but it did not occur often. It was caused by the multiple medications administered, including an allergic reaction to a medication being given that all turned toxic together, and the body could not expel the medications due to retaining excessive water. While in the hospital, I gained twenty to thirty pounds of fluid weight.

My legs look like tree trunks. My whole body was swollen. Once the doctors determined the problem, they started resolving it and treating it. Thank God, the delirium was only temporary. It took a while for me to return to my conscious state. Once the medication started to clear out of my system, I started to return to consciousness. I woke up. Hallelujah! The medical staff was amazed to see me talking and responding to them when they came to my room because they remembered my unresponsiveness. To them, it happened so rapidly. Ultimately, my return to a normal state happened slowly. It took a few weeks for me to feel, think, and physically like my old self.

Upon my discharge, all of these different doctors from various specialties came to my room. At the time, I did not know why so many doctors came to my room. I thought it was routine. However, it was because I was so sick. Each doctor was there because they treated a medical issue during my stay at the hospital. All the doctors came with their team of residents. I smiled politely as everyone came to the room.

Except for my primary doctor, all of the doctors asked you don't remember that I came to your room? When I said no, they looked with a slight surprise and smiled. Then they started talking to their residents about my condition. They knew I did not recall them coming to my room. I think they did it for training purposes. Every doctor had to give clearance before I could be discharged from the hospital. A nurse assistant stayed in my room 24 hours a day. My husband told me it was because I kept trying to get out of bed and fell more than once. I thought it was because I was so sick.

I could not do much for myself. She did not leave until the day before my discharge.

Leaving my room was one of the requirements for me to go home. I was so weak and scared to get out of bed. With the nurse's help, I went from bed to the chair. I stayed in the chair all day long. However, I had to prove that I could care for myself and walk.

Nonetheless, the nurses did not want me to leave the chair without first calling them. They did not know it, but I was too afraid to move. I was determined to get out of bed with little assistance. I wanted to go home. Home, I went the next day. When the primary doctor came to my room, I said, "I want to go home." Yes, it was time to go home. I was in the hospital long enough.

There is power in intercessory prayer. Intercessory prayer is simply praying for others. Continually, Jesus prays for us.

"For there is one God and one mediator between God and mankind, the man Christ Jesus... (1 Timothy 2:5, NIV)."

"He is sitting on the right hand of the Father interceding for us (Romans 8:34, NIV)" When I could not pray for myself, others were interceding for me. Others praying for me allowed for the will of God to happen, which was for my healing to come forth. No principality or power can stand against those who know how to pray. Intercessory prayer creates results and releases the supernatural power for victory to occur. It is a force that goes across the boundaries of time and moves the eternal power of God into your life and the lives of others.

As I said, I had others praying for me on one accord. *"If two of you shall agree on earth as touching anything they ask, it shall be done for them of my Father who is in heaven. For where two or three are gathered together in my name, there am I in the midst of them" (Matthew 18:19-20, ESV)."*

A pastor friend, Pastor Annie Brown, came to the hospital one night with some prayer warriors called Women Who Pray, and they drove around the hospital area seven times like the walls of Jericho interceding in prayer for me, sounding the alarm with the Shofar *(Joshua 6:2-17)*. In addition, they continuously prayed for me outside in the rain.

They believed that the strength and power of their prayers would cause my illness to vanish from my hospital room and restore my health completely. I would awaken with the same complete healing as when I arrived at the hospital—nothing missing or broken. Their requests were granted. Prayer possesses power. I am on my way to recovery and complete healing. Not only did they pray for me, but other people, some of whom I don't even know, were praying for me.

Warriors stood in the gap for God's will to be carried out. I recovered, thanks to the power of prayer.

Everyone who prayed for me deserves a special thank you from me to God's ears. Prayer has power, whether you believe it or not. I have faith.

Many people contemplating having a stem cell transplant have many questions. Some questions go from when to have a stem cell transplant to hospital stays. Length of stay and type of stem cell transplant. Questions, questions, and more questions. So many questions that the amyloidosis support group attempts to answer to the best of their knowledge. I had various questions, too, but I soon learned that everyone's experience differs. What happens to one person does not necessarily mean it will happen to you.

Like myself, my reaction to a stem cell transplant does not happen often. My experience is out of the ordinary.

Since the unexpected happened, I ended up being in the hospital longer than expected.

The hospital stay went from two weeks to almost one month. Just because this happened to me does not mean it will happen to you. Many people have stem cell transplants without incident. I mainly mentioned the stem cell experience to tell others that prayer is powerful. When you cannot pray for yourself, others are praying for you. Prayer is the only mechanism to influence and move God. It is your direct communication with Him. So, when a problem arises, pray and thank Him for answered prayer no matter how long it takes to manifest. Prayer stirs the atmosphere in the spirit realm. People reached out to God by faith through prayer seeking intervention from Him. I am the result of answered prayer. All things are possible if you can believe in God.

The day of my stem is considered my new birthday. It is a rebirth: a new life, a new beginning, a new start. The hospital has a birthday celebration for receiving your new stem cells. I received a birthday card and a cake for the celebration. Now, I have two birthdays, the day I was born and when I received my new stem cells. It is a celebration. I have a new life.

"Every experience in your life is another chapter added."
Martha Ehlert

Chapter 5

EMOTIONAL WHIRLPOOL

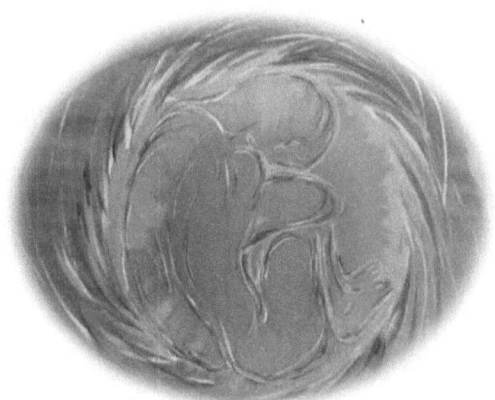

Steven Smith

Life is filled with constant change. One never knows when that change is going to come. Who knew a change was coming into the atmosphere that I could not reverse?

Things did not go according to plan, at least not as I had foreseen. In the beginning, I was not depressed. I thought my medical condition would be solved instantly with a simple diagnosis.

Run a few tests, take a pill, and the mystery will resolve itself. Just that simple. So, I thought. My life would return to normal as I knew it. After being told of my illness, I went from a happy and satisfied life to disbelief, shock, bewilderment, sadness, grief, anger, and fear. All of these emotions wrapped up into one. Eventually, acceptance of my new normal became a reality I had to overcome.

My emotional state went on a rollercoaster ride. Sometimes I was up, and then I was down. In the beginning, I was mostly down, very down. I was downright depressed. Looking at me, you would never know because I always kept smiling. I was going through an emotional turmoil on the inside. There were many times I did not feel very optimistic. I was wearing a mask that no one could see.

Those closest to me did not realize the fullest extent of my emotional turmoil. I was in a daze, just going through the motions. I felt isolated even though there were people around me, my immediate family, and close friends. I didn't think they could completely understand.

How could they? I did not entirely understand. I was in a cocoon looking from the inside out. I felt trapped. If you asked me how I felt, I would say I am okay or good. I was wearing an invisible mask, hiding behind my true feelings.

Think about going to the doctor and being told that you have a rare disease and cancer. There is no cure for either; the only way they can control it is with chemotherapy and/or stem cell transplant. Further, they can't tell you how long you will have to take chemotherapy.

The doctor answers that we will see how the treatment progresses. If you don't take chemotherapy, the disease can cause further and irreversible damage to your organs and body.

As a result of major organ damage, you could eventually die. I never imagined that I would ever have to do chemotherapy. Not in this lifetime. After all, there is no family history of cancer. No one in the family has ever heard of Amyloidosis. I have to do chemotherapy because I have a form of Multiple Myeloma and AL Amyloidosis.

Chemotherapy is the only mechanism to treat AL Amyloidosis/Multiple Myeloma. I have no choice. Let me say this we all have a choice. Either you do, or you don't. The choice of not doing anything was grim. At that point, my world fell apart. My feelings went from denial to anger, fear, and depression. You're thinking, let's start this conversation over with a different ending.

Usually, people discussing grief stages talk about someone who has died and/or in the process of dying. I feel that I went through what I call an emotional and spiritual death.

In some form, I went through some of the same stages to an extent. I was dying emotionally on the inside.

At first, I was in denial. I did not want to believe that this was happening to me. I saw it in some papers in my medical record but looked at it and could not fathom that written on the page was talking about me. I heard the doctor talking to me but wanted to deny everything the doctor told me.

Someone else must be in the room, and I overheard the conversation. Not me! How could this happen to me? I was not pretending that this was happening to me. I was trying to absorb and understand what was happening. My reality had shifted in a split second. I was in disbelief. It was taking my mind some time to adjust to my new reality.

According to Jodi Clarke (2020), denial attempts to slow the process of coping with new information as it takes individuals through one step at a time rather than risk the potential of feeling overwhelmed by emotions one is experiencing.

Once I went through the denial phase, then I got angry. Most of all, I got angry with God. Some people would never admit that they got mad with God. However, I am being honest, and as much as I know the scriptures that went out the window. I did not immediately go to my bible and search the scriptures. This was a huge mistake. I have no problem saying I got mad with God and wondered why this was happening to me. I asked, why was this happening to me? Why? Why? Why? The why's could not be answered. I did not get a response, or so I thought. I am sure God was speaking to me because He is always speaking. However, I was so upset and angry that I could not hear Him even when He spoke to me. God is always there, but I could not see and/or hear it.

I did not turn my back on God but was mad at Him. I could not talk or pray. I could not say a word. How could He allow this to happen to me? I thought I was faithful to the ways of God. I was active in ministry. I tried to rationalize why this was happening to me.

The bottom line is that bad things happen to good people. When I think about it, I feel I was going through a Job experience to some extent where God allowed certain things to happen to Job, but God told the devil he could not kill him. Months later, I received a word of encouragement from a lovely mother at a Women's Pray-fast and was told that this illness was not unto death, do not fear.

I never forgot the word of encouragement that was given to me, and I remember it to this day. Later I read scriptures to confirm the word given to me, *"This sickness is not unto death, but for the glory of God, that the Son of God may be glorified through it (John 11:4, NKJV)."* Initially, as I said in the beginning, I was angry with God. I was trying to adjust to a new reality. To encourage myself, I remembered, ***"Many of the afflictions of the righteous, but the Lord delivers him out of them all (Psalms 34:19, NKJV)."***

Next, I felt a sense of fear—the fear of the unknown. Fear paralyzes you and makes you immovable. All I could see was fear. At first, I thought I was going to die. I learned about my disease, and I thought the end was near. How near was the unknown? I went on google chrome and researched. The information appeared frightening, and fear started to set in. Some of the information went from bad to very bad. This was not good at all.

My initial visit with the doctor, to my next visit with the oncologist, was a few weeks away. I had a lot of time to ponder before receiving a final confirmation about my diagnosis. Fear and depression started to set in. The fear with the combination of depression was a mixture of disaster. It made everything worse. My thoughts were in a whirlwind. Because it is a rare disease, I needed to wait for an opening with an oncologist with expertise in Amyloidosis. Experts in the area of Amyloidosis are extremely limited.

There was only one doctor in my area whom other doctors and the Amyloidosis Support Group highly recommended. So, I had to wait. There was a considerable amount of time for fear to permeate my mind.

Lastly, I went into the depression stage. Depression robbed my hope. It killed my joy. It generated a heavy, oppressive feeling. Life looked bleak. Eventually, depression took over like a dark, heavy cloud. It drained every emotion like a plaque. This was when Satan came in for the attack.

He can come in unnoticed, silently, because your vision is blurred. You can't see anything other than what is in front of you.

All the negative images and thoughts flood your mind, and gloom and doom are in the midst. ***Your adversary, the devil, walks about like a roaring lion seeking whom he may devour (1 Peter 5:8, NKJV).*** He watches and comes in for the attack. As I said earlier, this is a rare disease, so there was no one I knew whom I could talk to except the doctor. I was a walking zombie. No one could identify with the way that I was feeling. I was going through the everyday motions. I felt isolated. At the time, I felt the church could not even help me, even though I knew many people in the Christian community. I did not know whom to reach out to or whom to talk to. My husband felt lost and did not know what to do. He didn't know what to say. He was extremely worried about me.

I spoke to my husband between the tears. He empathized with me but could not completely understand since he had never heard of the disease, nor did he expect this ever to happen. This is what I call life. One of the bumps in the road, and now I have to handle it.

For a long time, I wondered when it would be my turn for something good to happen. Have you ever experienced a time in your life when you wondered when it would be your turn? You watched from the outside, looking at everyone else's happiness, joy, healing, and success. Then, again, you question when it is my turn. An inkling of jealousy rouses up inside of your belly for a moment. Then soon goes away. Why them and not me?

My mind was barraged with negative thoughts. I did not think I was immune to sickness and disease. Most people, not all, at some point in their lives get sick.

I did not think the unexpected would happen now. Complaining was not going to change anything. Feeling sad was not going to alter anything. I have just to put one foot in front of the other, get up and keep it moving. Then I say, my turn is next.

"Through faith and patience inherit the promises of God (Hebrews 6:12, KJV)." As time passed by, a flicker of hope appeared.

I stood on the Word of God, remembering that I belonged to Him. By the stripes of Jesus, I am healed. He was wounded for my transgressions and bruised for my iniquities (Isaiah 53:5, NKJV).

Chapter 6

GAINING EMOTIONAL SUPPORT

Do Not Drown In Your Own Emotions. Take A Breather, Regain Your Strength, and Do Not Let What Worries, Control You.
Quotes Gate

In comes Amyloidosis Online Support Group, my initial lifeline. I needed someone to talk to, and I reached out to Muriel Finkel, the President of the Amyloidosis Online Support Group. Immediately, she called me back. I told her my story between the tears that she had heard so many times.

She was so comforting, patient, and understanding. She directed me to the online support group where patients and caregivers around the country can reach out to each other. Only patients diagnosed with Amyloidosis and relatives are part of the support group. The group provides awareness, information, and support, a shoulder to lean on in times of despair. Peer support group meetings are held with patients, caregivers, and doctors who are considered experts in treating Amyloidosis patients. Since I was diagnosed, I have had the opportunity to attend. They are very educational. Individuals can share their stories, and victories, and learn innovative and current treatments for the disease.

The online support group came when I needed someone the most. It did not answer all my questions, but it was a great help. The support group is a continued help to so many people. So many would be lost without it. It is a community.

Support groups are an effective means to help individuals that need help with various issues. It is a mechanism of survival for many people. Unfortunately, where I reside, local support groups are non-existent. I am grateful for the small personal contacts.

On my journey, I met my first Amyloidosis friend, who resides in Chicago. I reached out to her through the online support group. It was a blessing that she reached back to me.

It was nice to talk to someone who had the same diagnosis. I did not have to figure out the entire puzzle. I only had to understand a piece of the puzzle. As time went along, with a new piece of the puzzle came clarity. She comprehended everything I was feeling and saying. She could sympathize with my pain. It was a release. Even though we received different modes of treatment, the course of treatment and medication names were familiar to some extent. She had already been in the fight for over four years. Therefore, she was full of information and support. I had the pleasure of being able to meet her on a trip that she was taking. God had it that she had a stopover on the way to her cruise. I believe God places people in your life for a reason and a season.

She was placed in my life for such a time as this. To this day, she has been very supportive and is always there when I need support and information. Unfortunately, she resides too far away.

Nonetheless, we maintain frequent contact with each other. The friendship is mutual. I have met other people along the way. Unfortunately, none of the relationships are like the one I share with my Amyloidosis friend. Developing ongoing and close relationships is difficult due to the nature of the disease and distance. Most people do not reside in close proximity.

However, I have managed to meet some friendly people who reside not too far away. We attempt to meet each other for lunch occasionally to keep each other encouraged.

Speaking with other individuals diagnosed with Amyloidosis, experienced the same initial shock as I did.

After a while, I didn't give it a second thought that I needed professional help. I was depressed. I was at a loss and did not see how I would overcome the situation. I did not see the light at the end of the tunnel. Counseling was something that I had never considered in my life. I never thought that I would need counseling. Some individuals with Amyloidosis seek help continuously or sporadically during different points and times of treatment. Others none at all.

For me, talking through issues with a neutral party was essential. This was a person that was outside my circle of friends and family. I had no one that could understand what I was going through. I had no one that heard of the disease. They could not comprehend and/or imagine what I was experiencing. During the initial phase of my diagnosis, I saw a psychologist. Not that the psychologist understood my circumstances, but they are trained to listen to others without bias.

The psychologist helped me work through some of the issues I was facing. After reaching a certain point, I felt it was no longer effective. I talked, questions were asked, and I responded. For me, I solved my problems. I guess that is the purpose of visiting a psychologist. Counseling served its purpose. It took me to the next point where I could survive.

Even so, something was still missing. For me, it was a more profound spiritual component. I soon left, not to return.

My immediate family, specifically my husband, is a significant part of my Amyloidosis journey. He is the most important person in my care team because he is with me almost 24 hours daily and knows me better than any doctor.

Not only is he the most important person in my care team, but he is a huge part of my life.

I have been with my husband for over twenty-one years. He is my emotional support advocate. He has been with me every step of the way. When we found out about the diagnosis, I could see the despair on his face. He thought he was hiding it from me, but I saw it. When you have been with someone as long as we have been married, you can most of the time read the facial expressions.

Body language is more powerful than words. I am quite sure that secretly he wondered why this was happening to us, to me. He had to keep his faith in God, no matter the circumstances. He was worried as anyone would be. He felt helpless. This was a problem he could not solve. When men cannot solve problems, it brings a feeling of powerlessness.

Mainly, my husband being my sole caretaker was not easy.

The next phase of my treatment was dealing with a stem cell transplant. This meant he had to take time off from work and stay at home.

My stem cell transplant came at a time during COVID-19. Everything in society was mainly on lockdown. This meant he could not come to the hospital to visit.

My husband was unhappy that he could not visit every day, but that was the rule. We figured that we could use video chat to talk to each other. It provided some solace for both of us. Upon my release, he had to take me to all my doctor's appointments because I could not drive. I was too weak. It created moderate pressure having to take care of my daily needs until I gained enough strength for myself. When I came home from the hospital, he was nervous because he did not know what to expect.

However, he was a trooper and took everything in stride. I am sure my husband sometimes felt lonely, but he is a talker. Talking to others was a way of escaping and dealing with the circumstances.

When a spouse is very sick, the vows spoken at the marriage ceremony in sickness and health become very real. Not many couples can withstand the trial. I thank God for my husband standing next to me. I know people with the same illness and their husbands and/or partners could not withstand the test of time.

When Running Up A Hill, It Is all right To Give Up As Many Times You Wish-As Long As Your Feet Keep Moving On
Dan Millman

Chapter 7

SPIRITUAL PRESCRIPTION

Sometimes life hits you in the head like a brick. Don't lose faith.
Steve Job

The heart of prayer is asking God to intervene in matters concerning our daily lives. Remember, God gave man dominion over the things on earth. Therefore, we must pray to Him to handle our situations and circumstances. We cannot function to our fullest potential without God. It is His will that you and I be healed. It is not His will for us to be sick.

There is power in the prayer of the Word of God. When we pray, God's presence becomes a part of our prayers. The Word of God says, *"Let us, therefore, come boldly to the throne of grace, that we may obtain mercy and find grace to help in time of need." (Hebrews 4:16, NKJV)."*

When we pray, God hears us. We know we have what we ask of Him (1 John 5:15, NIV); whatever we ask of Him, you will receive it if you have faith (Matt 21:22, ESV)

I felt I had lost control of my life and needed help emotionally. The initial psychologist I was supposed to go to did not work out. This arrangement was made through the EEO program at my job. First of all, it took a long time for her to contact me. Next, when I spoke to the psychologist, convenient hours could not be agreed upon and would conflict with my job. Lastly, I did not get good vibes from the psychologist when we spoke on the phone. It was not a good fit. This was what I called God working behind the scenes for the correct intervention because the right psychologist was eventually located, the hours were convenient, and the psychologist was closer to home.

I firmly believe that if God is in the midst of something, He adds no sorrow. Religion could not be discussed during counseling sessions because of ethical boundaries. This is the protocol for most professions. However, in our conversations, I could tell she was a Christian because of the things she would reference in a roundabout way. Indirectly, she referred to God. I knew that I was placed in the right environment.

The psychologist was excellent but could not do what God could do. Everything has its limitations and purpose. You see, a psychologist can only go so far. God has to do the rest. I needed something more significant and potent than the psychologist could provide, which I called a spiritual prescription.

If you are sick, you go to the doctor to get healed. If you need counseling, you visit a therapist. You see an accountant and/or financial advisor if you need financial advice.

If you have a mental health problem, visit a psychologist and/or psychiatrist. Whatever you need in life, you visit an expert to help solve your problem. I was physically sick and mentally dying, so I needed spiritual healing. I needed spiritual medication. I needed help from the power of God, the type of healing that only God can do. Jesus said, *"Come to me, all of you who are weary and carry heavy burdens, and I will give you rest (Matthew 11:28, NKJV)."* God was not my enemy; he was not the cause of my illness. He is the mighty healer, Jehovah Rophe.

I knew there was a flicker of hope, love, and joy in the Word of God. I had to learn to fall back in love with Him as He never left me, the agape type of love. A love that emulates the love of God. God never stopped loving me for one moment. The power of the love of God is just like that.

Not everyone will acknowledge it, but I confess that I was mad at God, so I turned my back, trying to cope with reality.

I had to come to the realization that I could not do it alone. My help was just around the corner, waiting for me.

Only God could help me. I had to go from a place of darkness to light. After discovering my illness, I was in a very dark place for months. No one knew except me. I smiled every day and was crying on the inside. Tears that only God knew about. I needed a spiritual prescription. *God's Word strengthens the weary (Isiah 40:29, NKJV)*

> *"Hope is the inextinguishable flickering God ignites in our souls to keep us believing in the prevailing power of His light even when we are surrounded by utter darkness."*
> **Lee Strobel**

Flickering Light

I was lying in bed, in and out of sleep. The remote for the bed was lying in the middle of the bed. In and out of sleep, I noticed the light on the remote flicker. I looked at the remote again; a few minutes later, it flickered. I thought this was strange; I had never noticed that before. Then a few seconds later, it flickered one more time. Just as it started, then it suddenly stopped. I say the flickering of light represented hope in my life, a new life, my new normal. Darkness cannot comprehend the light. Darkness and light cannot stay in the same location. As long as there is light, there is always hope.

Provided I continue to believe and trust in God, hope always lingers in the atmosphere. It just takes a flicker of thought to move you in the right or wrong direction. So, Paul said, **"I pray that God, the source of hope, will fill you completely with joy and peace because you trust in him.**

Then you will overflow with confident hope through the power of the Holy Spirit (Romans 15:13, NLT)."

June of 2019 was the day I stepped out of the darkness into the marvelous light. My ministerial friends, Pastor Annie Brown and Rev. Christine Maxwell came to my home in a time of need and prayed with me. God always knows when to step in if you will allow Him. He uses other people to get His will done. When they came to my home, I invited God to handle my situation. They were God's mouthpieces. They prayed with me, gave me words of encouragement, and brought me a treasure chest full of herbs to assist with my health. Once they prayed with me, a weight started to lift off of my shoulders. God's presence took over. As long as you are living, there is always hope. *"Let us hold fast the confession of our hope without wavering, for He who promised is faithful" (Hebrews 10:23, NKJV).*

Biblical hope allows us to look away from a narrow perspective and opens us up to a larger view of faith in the expectation of receiving God's promises and extraordinary things.

Faith

There are many things in my life that I had to believe by faith, hoping that God would move on my behalf, and He did. Nothing has tested my faith to this magnitude more than believing God for my healing from a rare disease and cancer.

When you are confronted with major life events, this is when you know whether you are living by faith or if it is just words that you speak about. This is when faith steps in. *"Those who have faith and patience inherit the promises of God" (Hebrews 6:12, NKJV).*

Since my diagnosis, I have had a renewed perspective on faith. I always believed in God's Word and lived by faith.

Without faith, it is impossible to believe God (Hebrews 11:6, NKJV). When you are fighting literally for your life, hope and faith for healing magnifies in your life. Faith is the ingredient to things hoped for. Hope doesn't vacillate or get lost in circumstances because it is deep-rooted in the faithfulness of God. Hope is the sense of expectancy and optimism that God will move on an individual's behalf who has faith in Him. Even in the midst of our greatest problem, God is still with us. He is greater than any challenge we might face.

Faith is not about feeling and/or what can be seen. If you can see it and have it, you don't need faith. Faith is not about sight. It grabs hold of the unseen, not the seen. You have to believe that you already have it even though you cannot see it. Believe in your healing in the present and not the future because Jesus Christ has already completed the work. *The Son of Man came to destroy the devil's works (1 John 3:8, NIV), poverty, sickness, and disease; by his stripes, we were healed (1 Peter 2:24, NIV).* Since we were healed, we are healed.

Your faith is tested when you have an illness that can kill you. It takes faith to a whole new level and the meaning of what you think you believe. The Bible says, *"NOW faith is the assurance (title deed, confirmation) of things hoped for (divinely guaranteed), and the evidence of things not seen [the conviction of their reality—faith comprehends as fact what cannot be experienced by the physical senses] (Hebrews 11:1, AMP)."* Now meaning present tense. Faith is for NOW, not tomorrow. Jesus Christ has already done the work and continues to do it right now. Healing belongs to you and me.

"He personally carried our sins in His body on the cross (willingly offering Himself on it, as on an altar of sacrifice), so that we might die to sin (becoming immune from the penalty and power of sin) and live for righteousness; for by

His wounds you (who believe) have been healed (1Peter 2:24, AMP)." Healing belongs to everyone who believes in Jesus Christ. Believe that you have received your healing NOW. We all live in the NOW. So, believe in your NOW healing, not tomorrow healing. You have to speak the words of faith even when others are not.

Faith does not mean you don't use what God has made available in the earth realm. For instance, faith has nothing to do with not taking your medication and/or taking the doctor's advice. Take your medication, get advice from your doctors, and believe God by faith for your healing. You cannot blame God if you get sick from not taking your medication and/or blame the doctor if things are not working as you expect.

So, take your medication and follow the directions of the doctor. I have to admit that I have personally stopped and/or cut back on my medication.

When I go to the doctor, the first question is, are you taking your medication? If you lie, you are only hurting yourself. I tell the truth. Then I am told to take my medication.

Medication has nothing to do with your faith. Medication helps to deal with the symptoms until healing is manifested naturally. Faith is based on believing God for what you ask is received. Your healing is already operating in the spiritual realm. It just has to be manifested in the natural realm.

Doctors can only go to a certain point; God steps in by faith, and He does the rest. Healing comes from God and God alone. Frederick Price (1997) mentioned that God has already built healing in our bodies. Given all the parameters, the body will heal itself. Therefore, until healing occurs, confess the Word of God by faith, believing for the manifestation.

Do not lose faith. Know that God hears you. Why do we have faith in God? Because He never fails!

Daniel 10:12, Daniel did not lose faith because he felt his prayer was not answered immediately. The answer did not come until twenty-one days later. *"Then he said to me, do not fear, Daniel, for from the first day that you set your heart to understand and to humble yourself before your God, your words were heard, and I have come because of your words.*

But the prince of the kingdom of Persia withstood me twenty-one days (NKJV)" If Daniel gave up so easily the first day, his prayer would not have been answered. Keep the faith! Even if what you believe God for has not manifested when you think it should, KEEP THE FAITH! It is coming. Pray by faith, knowing you have already received your healing. Have faith in God.

Believe that what you say will come to pass. Have faith in God, the God kind of faith (Mark 11:22, NKJV). This means that when God spoke things, they came into existence (Genesis 1:3-26, NKJV).

If you are a child of God, you have the same characteristics. You carry His DNA. The Word of God says, *"Let us make man into Our own image, according to Our likeness and let them have dominion… (Genesis 1:3:26, NKJV)."* We have dominion and power over our healing. When you confess healing, believe it will also come to fruition. "For assuredly, I say to you, whoever says to this mountain (healing from cancer and Amyloidosis), be removed and be cast into the sea,' and does not doubt in his heart, but believes that those things he says will be done, he will have whatever he says. *"Therefore, I say to you, whatever you ask when you pray, believe that you receive them, and you will have them"* (Mark 11:23-24, NKJV)." Faith does not believe God can't but knowing He can and will. *"When you decree and declare a thing, it shall be established for you"* (Job 22:28, NKJV).

There are no buts, and it's in faith. Avoid anything contrary to the Word of God. *"Keep this Book of the Law always on your lips; meditate on it day and night so that you may be careful to do everything written in it. Then you will be prosperous and successful (Joshua 1:8, NIV)."* Don't look to the left or the right because you can get distracted.

At times, this is not easy due to outside factors and influences. I know because it happened to me. The moment I took my eyes off the Word of God, the devil stepped in and said I gotcha. I had to make a concentrated effort to keep my eyes on the Word of God.

Faith comes by hearing and hearing the Word of God (Romans 10:17, NKJV)." Hearing and hearing and hearing. Reinforce yourself with the Word of God. *"Put on the helmet of salvation and take the sword of the Spirit which is the Word of God (Ephesians 6:17, NLT)."* In addition,

"Take up the shield of faith with which you can extinguish all the flaming arrows of the evil one (Ephesians 6:16, NIV)."

Stand on the Word of God no matter what you feel or what comes across your mind. Just stand firm on the Word of God until you receive your breakthrough. Faith moves the hand of God. Faith accepts God's Word as final. Faith possesses the promises of God. Faith is not an option. It is a requirement. We all should live a life where faith exists.

Prayer
> *"Prayer is not asking. Prayer is putting oneself in the hands of God, at His disposition, and listening to His voice in the depth of our hearts."*
> ***Mother Teresa***

The heart of prayer is asking God to intervene in matters concerning our daily lives. Remember, God gave man dominion over the things on earth.

Therefore, we must pray to Him to handle our situations and circumstances. We cannot function to our fullest potential without God. It is His will that you and I be healed. It is not His will for us to be sick.

There is power in the prayer of the Word of God. When we pray, God's presence becomes a part of our prayers. The Word of God says, *"Let us, therefore, come boldly to the throne of grace, that we may obtain mercy and find grace to help in time of need." (Hebrews 4:16, NKJV)." When we pray, God hears us. We know we have what we ask of Him (1 John 5:15, NIV); whatever we ask of Him, you will receive it if you have faith (Matt 21:22, ESV).*

Prayer had to become my answer. I guess I had stopped praying because I felt God did not hear my prayers. For a long time, I lost heart to pray. When I opened my mouth, no words came to thought. I could not utter a word.

I was in a complete blink. My mind was clueless when it came to me. I did not know what to pray for. I was in spiritual warfare, a spiritual battle for my life. In the past, I prayed for everyone else and heard their praise reports. Why? Why not me, Lord? I felt helpless, forgetting that there is strength in prayer. I became distracted by my circumstances. This is how the devil comes in to destroy. ***The devil roams around like a roaring lion to see whom he may devour (1 Peter 5:8, NKJV).*** The devil plays for keeps, leaving nothing behind that comes in his pathway. I believed in Jesus, but I stopped believing in the power of my prayers. The Word of God says, ***"Resist the devil, and he shall flee from you (James 4:7, NKJV)."***

So, I ask, "Is prayer your steering wheel or spare tire (*Corrie Ten Boom*)?" Prayer is my steering wheel. It guides our life. Prayer is a powerful weapon. It is our defense mechanism. Don't let it become your spare tire.

When we start to pray, the devil gets nervous and starts to tremble. It is the best weapon that we know. Prayer is our connection to God. When we release prayer in the atmosphere, it starts working in the spiritual realm to bring forth fruit in the natural realm. It activates the movement of God. *God has commissioned his angels to watch over us and to keep us in all our ways (Psalms 91:11, NKJV).*

I had to go back to God in prayer. Only God knows how many tears I cried and how many prayers I initiated in my secret place that only He heard. *The Father who sees what is done in secret will reward you (Matthew 6:6, NIV).* I had to believe and trust God by faith that when I pray, God hears me. If I know that he hears me, whatever I ask, I know that I have whatever I asked of Him, and healing is His will.

Remember, we must invite God to intervene on our behalf, which is called prayer.

God gave man dominion over everything on earth, so we must walk in the power and authority He gave us. Life and death lie in the power of our tongue. The Word says I will give you keys to the Kingdom.

"Whatever you bind on earth will be bound in heaven, and whatever you loose on earth will be loosed in heaven. If two of you agree on earth concerning anything that they ask, it will be done for them by My father in heaven (Matt 18:18-19, NIV)." "For where there two or three are gathered in my name, I am there in the midst of them (Matt 18:20, NIV). Lastly, God says, when you call on Me and come and pray to Me, I will listen to you (Jeremiah 29:12, NKJV). God answers to prayer. As the saying goes, He may not come when you want Him, but he comes right on time.

Let's Pray Together

Today I come to you to confess the Word in the name of Jesus of Nazareth concerning healing over every disease plaguing the earth. In the name of Jesus of Nazareth, according to your Word, you sent your Word, and it will accomplish everything you sent it to do and will not return void. Therefore, in the name of Jesus of Nazareth, every person is healed of sickness and disease. Every symptom will not be tolerated and must leave and return from which it came in the name of Jesus of Nazareth. It is cut off at the root. You are Jehovah Rophe, The Lord Who Heals, and healing is according to your Word and will. Every promise is yes and amen. You are the mighty physician, so what doctors cannot do, you can do by faith. In the name of Jesus of Nazareth, I pray that God steps in and heal those who are sick in their homes and lying in hospital beds.

Restore their bodies to complete wholeness that is under attack. I declare and decree divine healing over respiratory systems, immune disorders and systems, blood disorders and systems, gastrointestinal disorders, cardiovascular systems, heart disease, neurological disorders, bone and spinal disease and deterioration, eye disorders, cancer of all types, and any organ failure in the name of Jesus of Nazareth. Every organ and tissue will function in the perfection that God created it to function. According to your word in *3 John*, we may prosper in all things and be healthy just as our soul prospers.

Now I plead the blood of Jesus of Nazareth over your people for their protection. Protect those who are in harm's way. Protect your first responders, nurses, and doctors and keep them from any sickness and/or illness that may attempt to come their way as they help others. When the enemy sees the blood, he must pass without a shadow of a doubt, as in the days of Moses. I bleed the blood of Jesus of Nazareth over our homes, our families, our friends, and our neighbors.

I speak to Satan and all his operations in the name of Jesus of Nazareth that your principalities, powers, spirits who rule in darkness, and spiritual wickedness in heavenly places are bound from operating against God's Word and people in any manner. Every unclean spirit must flee in the name of Jesus of Nazareth. Remove yourself and go back from the gates that you have entered. We are the property of the Almighty God, and you have no authority over God's people. We abide stable and fixed under the shadow of the Almighty God whose power no foe can withstand. The kingdom of heaven has been subject to violence, and we take it back by force.

In the name of Jesus of Nazareth, every chain is broken off every person's life, poverty, sickness, and disease. Jesus came so the works of the devil might be destroyed and that we might have life and life more abundantly. Your word says in Gal 3 that Christ has redeemed us from the curse of the law, having become a curse for us. The prayers of the righteous are powerful and effective.

So, therefore, I come knocking on Your door. In your Word, if I ask, it shall be given to me. Seek, and I shall find, knock, and it will be opened to me. Father, I come to you expecting an open door of healing and the door has been opened for me to walk thru. My healing is in the midst of the atmosphere that has no boundaries. I call out to the North, South, East, and West winds for restoration, replenishment, and rejuvenation. Blow abundantly and profusely into my life without any hindrance or hesitations. No weapon formed against me shall prosper. I stand on your Word, believing and trusting in only you. Everyone who asks receives, and he who seeks finds, and to him who knocks, it will be opened.

I thank you, Father, for the open doors of healing and protection that only you can give. I declare and decree victory. I have the victory that overcomes the world. No power can withstand your Word and every knee must bow. Victory is mine in the name of Jesus of Nazareth. I walk in the power and love of God. His glory shines upon my life. He is forever present in my life, and I fear not. He has given me the mind of power, love, and a sound mind.

You are Jehovah Rophe, The God who heals; You are all-powerful; You are El Shaddai, God Almighty. You are the Lord of breakthrough, Jehovah Baal–Perazim. You are the ever-present God, Jehovah Shammah. You are the all-knowing God, the One who will never leave or forsake me. I thank you for all these things in the precious name of Jesus of Nazareth.

I thank you for what you have done in the past, what you have done in the present, and what is coming in the future in the name of Jesus of Nazareth. Amen

Remember, there is nothing that God cannot do because He is God and God alone. All things are possible if you can trust and believe by faith. We can expect a miracle because the power of His Word causes us to believe in answered prayer.

"Prayer should be the key of the day and the lock of the night."

- George Herbert

Chapter 8

TAKING CONTROL

Take Control of Your Life, Your Health, and Your Happiness
Meagan J. Spence

Getting the medical diagnosis is a scary experience. I did not know what to expect or the outcome. It was a complete surprise. The diagnosis impacted the rest of my life. My husband and I were devastated as we sat in the doctor's office. Therefore, I had to get all the information I could understand.

Before my appointment, I had written several questions, about fifteen or more. You may say that was a lot, but I had to ensure everything was covered. I considered myself to be well prepared. Some of the information I had read gave me the ability to know what the doctor was explaining and which questions to ask the doctor. In addition, the doctor saw I did my homework to explore my condition, which changed the tone of the doctor's visit, an informed patient versus a non-informed patient. Being informed about Amyloidosis helped me take control of my life, making it easier to discuss treatment options with my doctor.

We are responsible for our health. How often have we gone to the doctor and accepted everything without exploring the situation? It is our responsibility to take control of our health.

Finding a doctor can be problematic and finding the right doctor to accommodate all your specific needs can be downright confusing. When visiting the doctor, ensure you get a complete picture of your medical diagnosis and treatment options. Do not be afraid to ask questions until you get your desired response. Let me make it clear, get a thorough understanding. Some doctors tend to give medical terminology you don't understand. You are not in the medical field.

Don't settle until you get an understanding. *"In all thy getting get understanding (Proverbs 4:7 KJV)."* I don't think doctors intentionally mean to explain things in medical terminology. It is because they do it so often that it becomes second nature to them. They think you understand when you don't. Just think, each profession has a terminology that belongs explicitly to that profession, for example, child welfare, business organizations, computer technology, law enforcement, financial services, and the list goes on and on.

Only people on the inside of the profession are familiar with what the person is truly talking about. An outsider does not understand unless it is explained. Your medical history must be treated and understood in the same manner. It could mean life or death. If you don't get it, ask questions. After all, it is your body.

Get a second opinion if you don't like what you are hearing. **IF NECESSARY, CHANGE DOCTORS**. The main goal is to be healthy to the best of your ability.

This means mentally, physically, and emotionally. It would help if you grasped your doctor's recommendations about your medical condition. These are some of the questions I asked as I went along on my journey, including the responses.

What caused the disease? Unknown. Only between 4,000 to 5,000 people get it in a year in the USA

What is the prognosis, long or short-term? The disease was detected early, so the outcome was favorable. Remission is the long-term objective. The term "remission" can be easily understood.

What are the symptoms of the disease that I have? There were many that I mentioned.

When do I have to take laboratory tests? When do I get the results, and what do they mean? I would take labs weekly. The complete set of labs will be reviewed at a four-week interval with the doctor.

Why did I get Amyloidosis? In my situation, is it hereditary? There are various types. My type is not hereditary.

What are the risk factors of the disease and treatment? If treatment was not received immediately, the disease could further affect the organs, my condition could get worse, and it could be fatal in the future.

Are there any risk factors that are preventable and addressable? At the time of diagnosis, there were no preventable risk factors. It just happened.

The cause was unknown. The only way to address the issue was to have chemotherapy.

How will the disease impact me over the short and long term? Over the short term, without treatment, my condition would get worse. With treatment, my condition should hopefully get better over the long term. TIME WILL TELL

How is the disease treated? Is this the only way? What are my options? My only option was chemotherapy. TIME WILL TELL

How well will the chemotherapy work? It is expected that chemotherapy should go well.

Why do I need this treatment? This is the only option. Research has shown there are no other treatments except stem cell transplants. At this time, I am not eligible for a stem cell transplant. Recipients must meet stringent guidelines. My blood result numbers are too high.

The goal is obtaining remission through chemotherapy without considering a stem cell transplant. There are medical trials for some, but that is not an option the doctor chooses to take.

Further, my condition was not at that stage. There are various qualifications for medical trials. Some work, and some don't.

Why might someone consider delaying or not having treatment? This was not in my case. Not having treatment could potentially be fatal down the road.

How long will I need to take chemotherapy? Treatment varies with each individual, depending on the condition. Based on my diagnosis, I would receive chemotherapy treatment every four weeks for a minimum of 4 months. Then, depending on the outcome, a decision will be made to explore the next step.

When will chemotherapy stop? Chemotherapy will stop depending on the outcomes. TIME WILL TELL

How would chemotherapy help? This is the only way to reduce the amyloid in the body and/or stop further production, harming my body and causing irreversible damage.

Where will I be treated? Primary, I will be treated at an outpatient clinic. However, I will have to go to the hospital in case of an emergency or an unexpected medical condition arises.

You can ask your doctor these same questions to obtain as much information as needed, including more. I hope these are insightful and helpful.

I received a lot of information about my condition. At first, I did not understand all of the information given to me. I was not afraid to ask additional questions.

I continue asking questions today to understand what is happening to me completely. As I went along, I had additional questions.

Fortunately, I do not have a doctor who does not mind answering any questions I might have. Do not be afraid to take notes. If available, get resources, materials, brochures, and access reputable online medical organizations with viable information. I belong to an online support group that has not only helped with providing information but has information about other medical resources.

Choosing a doctor is like socializing. You hold the same values, see eye to eye and be on the same page regarding expectations. Most importantly, I had to find the right doctor. Choosing the right doctor was important to my health care.

Upon my diagnosis, I was advised to see a specialist who dealt with Amyloidosis patients and is the top in the field of

Amyloidosis. At first, I went to a hematologist/oncologist who knew about Amyloidosis, but he was not known to specialize in the area of my disease.

Nonetheless, he appeared to be a good doctor, but I decided to change. When he discovered that I wanted to change doctors, he initially refused to see me and provide test results that I waited two weeks to receive. My husband and I were irritated by his unprofessionalism. However, he hesitantly gave me the results after I insisted on getting my results.

Finally, based on the response that I received from the doctor, gave me confirmation to change my doctor. I made the correct decision and did not regret it one moment.

The doctor I now have was recommended by other doctors and the online support group I belong to. I am so elated that I did. I am proud to say his name is Dr. James Hoffman from the University of Miami.

It was the best decision that I had made about my health. Finally, I have a doctor who is concerned about me. He is patient, understanding, and knowledgeable, and he takes the time to ensure that I comprehend every step and the reasons for making decisions.

Dr. Hoffman investigated my medical history before my office visit. I was amazed that the doctor had my medical history before our initial meeting. He took the time to look at medical records that were readily available and obtained information from other hospitals. The doctor makes me feel as if I am his only patient. I never feel rushed out the door so that he can see his next appointment.

Most importantly, he gives me hope. He is passionate about his profession. When you are given a life-threatening condition for which there is no known medical cure, you need a doctor that can give you hope for the future. Further, to let you know that you will live and not die. This is what my doctor did, and I am forever grateful. I thank God for my doctor. He operates with compassion toward his patients. All of his patients express the same sentiment.

Qualities of a Good Doctor:
- Professionalism
- Display a sense of passion
- Empathic to your needs
- Knowledgeable
- Work Ethics
- Dedicated to the profession
- Confident
- Humility
- Keeps up to date with innovative new medical treatments

Chapter 9

FUTURE RECOMMENDATIONS

"Surround yourself with dreamers and doers, believers, and thinkers.
Most of all, surround yourself with those who see greatness in you."
Felicia Mabuza-Suttle on Twitter

Stay away from pessimistic people who have nothing good to stay, regardless of the situation. They can find fault and doubt in everything. There is a problem to every solution.

They carry a harmful spirit and attempt to push their negativity on you. On the whole, they are not happy about themselves. How could someone be so negative all the time and be happy? The answer is that they are not. Ignore them.

Do not allow a lack of enthusiasm and hopelessness in your immediate surroundings. Act like they do not exist. Do not accept phone calls, do not allow them to visit, and do not allow them to come in contact with you at all. You take their voice away when you do not allow negative people to invade your space. It inhabits somewhere else, and they can do nothing but eventually go away. Do yourself a gigantic favor and let go of people who are toxic to your life. You do not need naysayers around when you are fighting to restore your health. Please do not allow them to impact your present circumstances and surroundings. Negative people bring your spirit down and place discouraging thoughts in your mind. Negativity is like poison.

I canceled out all negativity. Negativity had no place in my life. I did not feel bad about it. It was important for my physical and mental health. Stress, tension, and unhappiness can kill you in the long term. It affects your body, and you don't think about it. One day, I had a relative that made me so upset that I immediately felt sick.

Since I was still under the doctor's care, at that point, I knew there were people that I needed to remove from my life. Other people's problems cannot be my problem. This includes family and friends. I cut that relative off without hesitation.

Have a positive support network that includes family and friends. Stay with optimistic people who believe the same way you believe and can uplift your spirit in a time of need. Good things happen when you change your environment.

When you experience a major health crisis and/or event in your life, you will encounter highs and lows. Hopefully, there will be more highs than lows. When I was feeling down, I always had someone who would have something positive to say to keep me encouraged. It would help if you had as much positivity around you as possible. For example, church, encouraging friends and relatives, professional counseling, significant other and/or husband. Whatever works for you, do it because that is your medicine and lifeline.

Meditate on positive things to overcome challenges you will undoubtedly encounter during your journey with your illness. Good mental health helps you to get through your day-to-day activities. When you have good mental health, it gives you clarity and keeps you focused. A healthy mental attitude allows you to make sound decisions about how you relate to others in your life and meet the new demands in your life.

Another interesting way to give stability is to write a journal, either handwritten or video. It was a good output for me. I have several journals around the house to place my thoughts. Secondly, I read books that interest me. Reading allows me to concentrate on other things. This included not looking at the news or any depressing shows on television.

The Food Network and HGTV and I became friends. Due to the coronavirus and stem cell transplant, I had to stay home. I found these stations to be relaxing.

I listened to spiritual music that gave inspirational messages. Inspirational music and sermons positively influence your mindset. It helps to boost your mood and reduce stress. Listening to inspirational music and sermons are powerful tools to promote overall health. Constantly, the devil attempts to invade your ear gate with fear and hopelessness. Hearing about a life-threatening disease is devastating. For me, inspirational music assisted me in reinforcing that God is in control. I will believe in the report of the Lord that I am healed.

I took quiet time for myself. This was very important. If you have the ability, take time to travel. I say GO without hesitation.

A change of atmosphere places you in a different mind frame. Do things that you like no matter what it is. If you cannot travel, do things locally, visit the park, restaurant, movies, botanical gardens, museum, etc. Enjoy your hobbies. It is VITAL for your stability and strength. Tomorrow is not promised to anyone, so live each day to the fullest.

We tend to take life for granted. The Bible says that life disappears quickly. *"Yet you do not know (the least thing) about what may happen in your life tomorrow. (What is secure in your life?) You are merely a vapor (like a puff of smoke or a wisp of steam from a cooking pot) that is visible for a little while and then vanishes (into thin air) (James 4:14, AMP)."*

This means that life is moving quicker than we can see or think. It is here today and gone tomorrow. Things change quickly. No matter what is occurring in your life, enjoy it to the fullest. I cannot stress the importance of taking hold of your life and enjoying the things that matter the most.

Tomorrow is not promised and/or guaranteed to anyone. One day I went to sleep healthy, and when I woke up, I was sick. My life changed forever, never to be the same again. I am living my new reality. I focus on what is important to me, which helps me to feel better.

Revaluate what is important in life, not allowing insignificant things to bother you. The way you view your life molds your life. Our perspective has everything to do with how we invest our time and whom we associate with in a social and personal arena. Ask yourself, how do you view where you are in life? According to life circumstances, the answer varies. We are here for a purpose. It is not over until God says it is over.

We are made a blessing to be a blessing to others. God has given us gifts and talents to utilize on this earth. We have God-given abilities to share with others.

Ultimately, it is for us to make a difference in this world. It is not about how long we live but how we have lived here on earth. My goal is to completely fulfill God's purpose and leave this life empty leaving an inheritance.

Healing does not always happen instantaneously. For many, healing happens over time. *"And these signs will follow those who believe in My name…they will lay hands on the sick and recover (Mark 16:17-18, NKJV)."* The word recover means to make progress (progression). Recovery means going from the point of being sick to the point of being healed. Again, healing does not happen overnight for everyone.

Having faith is imperative. KEEP THE FAITH. You cannot move without having some form of faith. Everyone is given a degree of faith, from little to great faith. Faith of a mustard seed can move God. Develop and strengthen your faith. *"Faith comes by hearing the Word of God (Romans 10:17, NKJV)."*

Some medical conditions take more faith than others. Healing depends on your faith level. The more you strengthen your faith, the more you can believe God for your healing. It is easier to believe God for a common cold than believe God for healing from a serious illness such as cancer. Therefore, strengthen your faith by reading and listening to the Word of God. Do not sit around waiting, calling it faith. This is not faith. This is foolishness. Build your faith. *"Faith without works is dead (James 2:17, NKJV)."*

Are you going to accept the help that God is sending your way? I have often heard this anecdote about a man sitting on top of a roof waiting for help due to a catastrophic flood. He prayed to God for help. God sent help three times by sending a man with a jet ski, a boat, and a helicopter to carry him to safety. Every time the man said that he was waiting on God for help. God is going to send me help. Eventually, the flood waters rose, and the man died. When the man went to heaven, he asked God what had happened. God told him, I sent you help three times, but you denied Me. An individual can have all the faith in the world, but without works faith is dead.

There was no corresponding action to faith. Faith and action must work hand in hand.

We are often given a head start on our sickness to initiate taking action, but we decide to wait with possible bad information and/or advice from what other people think we should do. *"First seek the Kingdom of God and His righteousness and all these things will be added to you" (Matt 6:33, NJKV).*

As an alternative, God sends help in the form of a doctor. If God did not want doctors in the earth realm, they would not be here. In the bible, Luke was a doctor. Doctors serve a purpose. The key is finding a good one.

I decided not to sit around and call it faith. Sometimes if you wait too long, you can worsen the medical condition to the point of no return. We serve a God that nothing is impossible for those who believe. Whatever decision concerns your health, make sure it is an informed decision.

Speak life. God has empowered us to speak life into every situation in our lives. *Death and life are in the power of our tongue. (Proverbs 18:1, KJV).* Our words are powerful and dynamic.

Our words create a force in the universe to be reckoned with. Words affect our destiny. Words form things that are in the present and future. Therefore, we cannot speak what we see but speak things that we hope for in the present and future. Everything we say shapes our life. So, it is imperative that we are careful about what we say. We may not feel or see it the minute we speak it, but those words are planting seeds, taking root.

Our words form our confession of what we believe and do not believe. In times of illness, we must confess what the Word of God promises about our healing. It is not about just speaking but believing what we desire by faith. *We walk by faith and not by sight (Romans 10:17, NKJV).*

So shall My word be that goes forth from My mouth; It shall not return to Me void, But it shall accomplish what I please, And it shall prosper in the thing for which I sent it,

Isaiah 55:11

Deposit good thoughts and good moments in your life. Things are not as bad as they seem or could be worse. Remember, things may not be great, but someone is not doing as well as you, trying to survive the next day. Good thoughts never produce bad results. Evil thoughts never produce virtue. Try to deposit positive thoughts in your mind continually. Negative thoughts tear you down mentally. They create worry and frustration. Don't let negative thoughts take over. I am not saying that it is easy but try. Count your blessings. Recall the many good things and be thankful.

The hardest thing to do is not to talk about your health. People call you and ask how you feel. We tend to talk about how we are feeling. According to David Schwartz (1959), talking about being unhealthy is like putting fertilizer on weeds. The more you talk about it, the worse you feel. Refuse to talk and worry about your health. Let the conversation be minimal and move to the following conversation with something more jovial. Talk about something that makes you smile. Life is yours to take pleasure in, so be happy.

Life is like a game of chess.

To win, you have to make a move.

Knowing which move to make comes with IN-SIGHT and knowledge, and by learning the lessons that are accolated along the way.

We become each and every piece within the game called life!"

Allan Rufus, The Master's Sacred Knowledge

CONCLUSION

It's Called Life

"If you want to conquer the anxiety of life, live in the moment, live in the breath."

Amit Ray, Om Chanting and Meditation

We never know what life is going to bring us. Life is full of ups and downs. We must handle it as it comes along. No one is exempt from grief or insulated from pain, illness, sickness, or disease. No one gets to glide through life without any problems. **"Many are the afflictions of the righteous, but God delivers him out of them all (Psalms 34:19, NKJV)."** Life is a deck of cards. We never know the deal that is dealt to us.

Unfortunately, every time you solve a problem, another comes along. They come in all shapes and forms. **Psalms 34:18 (NLT) says, "The Lord is close to the brokenhearted; he rescues those who are crushed in spirit."** When an individual such as myself suffers from an illness that cannot be cured, all you can depend on is God. God is all that you have and all you need. The doctors can only take you to a certain point, and you have to believe God to do the rest. Warren (2002) mentioned that none of our problems happens without God's permission. Everything that occurs to a child of God is Fathered-filtered, and He aims to use it for good even when Satan and others mean it for evil.

Despite all the obstacles, refuse to sit back and relax, letting life happen. Take control even though it may be difficult at times. Just believe by faith that help is coming your way. *"I know the plans I have for you," declares the Lord, " to prosper you and not to harm you, plans to give you hope and a future." (Jeremiah 29:11, NIV).* Everything that happens has some spiritual meaning. *"We know that God causes everything to work together for the good of those who love God and are called according to his purpose for them.*

God knew his people in advance and chose them to become like his Son" (Romans 8:28-29, NIV).

Adjust your attitude on life, and your outward life will change. You are the maker of your life.

We have the ability to conquer everything that is placed before us. *"No temptation has overtaken you except what is common to mankind. And God is faithful; he will not let you be tempted beyond what you can bear. But when you are tempted, he will also provide a way out so that you can endure it" (1 Corinthians 10:13, NIV).* Take the word impossible from your vocabulary. When you look at the word impossible, possible is inside the word. Impossible is a failure word. Possible is a word for success, encouragement, and achievable. Everything is possible if you can believe and trust that you are healed. No matter how you are feeling. Your body is aching, telling you something different.

The doctor's reports are saying what you do not want to hear. You can't go by how you feel, what you are told, and what you see. You have to go by what you believe in your heart by faith. From the heart, it goes to the mind, from the conscious to the subconscious mind. If you go by how you feel, your feelings will tell you contrary to I am healed.

"Above all else, guard your heart, for it is the wellspring of life" (Proverbs 4:23, NIV).

Believe until the end. **Where there is darkness, God has declared there to be light (Genesis 1:3).**

Every day, every minute, and every second is significant. Every day that I wake up is a blessing. I try not to take it for granted. We all have a lot to live for to the glory of God.

I have a testimony waiting to be told, and so do you. My testimony is how the goodness of God has made a difference in my life. I am a walking testimony.

This is now my New Normal. He has allowed me to live a victorious life. I continue to believe God for my complete healing every day, knowing that disease and sickness do not have any control over my body. If you can believe, God's promises are there for you to receive. It is not God's will for you to be sick. Sickness and disease do not glorify God.

I want you to believe that this is the dawning of a new day. Every day you are given is a new day for something fantastic to happen. Keep Believing! One day what you believe will come to pass.

The Essence Of A New Day

This is the beginning of a new day
You have been given this day to use as you will.
You can waste it or use it for good.
What you do today is important
Because you are exchanging a day of your life for it.
When tomorrow comes, this day will be gone forever.
In its place is something that you have left behind.
Let it be something good.
Author Unknown

Take advantage of today. Take advantage of tomorrow. As long as there is breath in our body and we wake up every day, there is hope. As long as we are breathing, we can make it.

God did not give you or me this illness. However, through my challenge with this illness, I can encourage someone else. You can make it one step at a time. Keep getting up no matter how you feel. When life knocks you down, get back up. God has us when we fall. He will grab and pick us back up when we are too weak to get up. When He picks us up, He is carrying us and walking for us, carrying us through. Stay strong and be of good courage. This is my journey. I walk it with victory in the mist. I have a purpose. This is my life. It is called life.

Today, I am in "complete response," some might call remission, to make it easier to understand. Tomorrow, I do not know what life will bring. So, I live each day to the fullest. I take the good with the bad. I do not sweat the small stuff. Trouble does not always last. It will soon pass. It is just a season. As long as my eyes open each day, there is tomorrow.

HEALING SCRIPTURES

Just believe, trust, and know that you are already healed. Healing is a promise from God. It is God's will to heal you. God can do abundantly above all we can ever ask, think, or imagine (Ephesians 3:20, NKJV).

Psalms 30:2 (NKJV) – *"O Lord my God, I cried out to you, and you healed me."*

Mark 9:23 (NLT) - *"Anything is possible if a person believes."*

Luke 17:19 (NLT) - *..." Your faith has healed you."*

3 John 1:2 (NKJV) - *"Beloved, I pray that you may prosper in all things and be in health, just as your soul prospers."*

1 Peter 2:24 (NKJV) – *"Whom Himself bore our sins in His own body on the tree, that we, having died to sins, might live for righteousness. By whose stripes you were healed."*

Psalms 91: 10-11 (NKJV) - *No evil shall befall you, Nor shall any plague come near your dwelling; For He shall give His angels charge over you, To keep you in all your ways.*

Psalms 103:3 (NKJV) – *"Who forgives all your iniquities, heals all your diseases."*

Psalms 107 19-20 (NIV) - *Then they cried to the L*ORD *in their trouble, and he saved them from their distress. He sent out his word and healed them; he rescued them from the grave.*

Matthew 17:20 (NKJV) *– "So Jesus said to them, "Because of your unbelief; for assuredly, I say to you, if you have faith as a mustard seed, you will say to this mountain, 'Move from here to there,' and it will move; and nothing will be impossible for you."*

Mark 11:23-24 (NKJV) *– "For assuredly, I say to you, whoever says to this mountain, 'Be removed and be cast into the sea,' and does not doubt in his heart, but believes that those things he says will be done, he will have whatever he says. Therefore, I say to you, whatever things you ask when you pray, believe that you receive them, and you will have them."*

Hebrews 13:8 (NKJV) *– "Jesus Christ is the same yesterday, today, and forever."*

Mark 21:22 (NLT) *– "You can pray for anything, and if you have faith, you will receive it."*

Psalms 30:2 (NKJV) – *"O Lord my God, I cried out to You, and You healed me."*

Matthew 7:7 (NKJV) – *"Ask, and it will be given to you; seek, and you will find; knock, and it will be opened to you."*

John 14:13 (NKJV) – *"And whatever you ask in My name, that I will do, that the Father may be glorified in the Son."*

Hebrews 10:23 (NKJV) – *Let" us hold fast the confession of hope without wavering for He who promised is faithful."*

Philippians 4:19 (NLT) – *"And this same God who cares for me will supply all your needs from His glorious riches, which have been given to us in Christ Jesus."*

Psalms 34:19 (NKJV) – *"Many are the afflictions of the righteous, but the Lord delivers him out of them all."*

Hebrews 4:16 (NKJV) – *"Let us, therefore, come boldly to the throne of grace, that we may obtain mercy and find grace to help in the time of need."*

Galatians 6:9 (KJV) – *Let us not grow weary while doing good; for in due season we shall reap if we faint not."*

Job 22:28 (NKJV) *– "You will also declare a thing, and it will be established for you."*

James 5:16 (NIV) *– "Therefore confess your sins to each other and pray for each other so that you may be healed. The prayer of a righteous person is powerful and effective."*

James 5:14 (NIV) *- Is anyone among you sick? Let them call the elders of the church to pray over them and anoint them with oil in the name of the Lord.*

*Nowhere in the Bible was a person not healed. God is no respecter of persons **(Acts 10:34, KJV)**. What was done for one, He will be done for another. Whoever asked for healing was healed by Jesus Christ. Healing did not stop with the death of Jesus. By the stripes of Jesus, we were all healed. The redemptive work was already done. God's Word is the same as yesterday, today, and forever **(Hebrews 13:8)**. Ask by faith. According to His Word, God does not lie **(Numbers 23:19)**. He sent His word, and it will accomplish what it was sent to do. Anything that we ask in the name of Jesus of Nazareth will be done. Go get your healing. It belongs to you. God Bless*

THANK YOU

Thank you to all the medical professionals at the University of Miami/Sylvester Cancer Center who continue to help me through this process. I am always greeted with a smile and a show of concern for my health. They helped to make a challenging process a little easier. The doctors, Dr. James Hoffman, Dr. Lazaros Lekakis, nurses, and other staff are special people. Everyone is not able to do their type of job daily. Yet, they continue to smile and give the gift of hope and life.

Also, I am grateful for my primary doctor, Dr. Rotem Amir, who was instrumental in helping to locate the diagnosis. Her persistence will always be remembered. They are a form of hope and encouragement that is needed daily. They are a gift to the medical community. No one wants to hear that you have cancer and/or a rare disease such as mine as Multiple Myeloma and Amyloidosis. I am forever grateful.

BIBLIOGRAPHY

Alsina, M. (2021). *Treatment Updates: Multiple Myeloma.* https://www.lls.org/sites/default/files/National/USA/Pdf/Slides_Transcipts/transcript_myeloma_3.2.21.pdf

American Cancer Society (2021). *Key Statistics About Multiple Myeloma.* https://www.cancer.org/cancer/multiple-myeloma/about/key-statistics.html

American Cancer Society (2020). *About Multiple Myeloma.* American Cancer Society. www.cancer.org/ content/ dam/CRC/PDF/Public/8738.00.pdf.

Amyloidosis Foundation (2020). *AL Amyloidosis.* Amyloidosis Foundation. www.amyloidosisfoundation.org

Amyloidosis: Statistics (January 2020). Cancer.Net. Editorial Board. https://www.cancer.net/ cancer-types/amyloidosis/statistics

Badii, C. (2019). *What's delirium, and how does it happen?* Healthline. Retrieved from https://www.healthline.com/health/delirium

Bible Gateway (n.d.). *Passage search.* Bible Gateway. https://www.biblegateway.com/

Bible Hub (2004-2020). *Online Bible Study Suite.* Bible Hub. https://biblehub.com/

Brenner, A. (2011). *The nature of change finds the predictable in the unpredictable. Psychology Now.*

https://www.psychologytoday.com/us/blog/in-flux/201105/the-nature-change-0

Cedars-Sinai (2019). *Amyloidosis*, Cedars-Sinai. www.cedars-sinai.edu/Patients/Health-Conditions/Amyloidosis.aspx.

Christian Veterinary Mission (2018). *Hope the inextinguishable flicker*. Christian Veterinary Mission. https://cvm.org/new-post/hope-vs-expectations/

Clarke, J. (2020). *The five stages of grief: Learning about emotions after a loss can help us heal.* https://www.verywellmind.com/five-stages-of-grief-4175361

Francis, J. (2020). *Delirium and acute confusional states: Prevention, treatment, and prognosis.* Retrieved from https://www.uptodate.com/contents/delirium-and-acute-confusional-states-prevention-treatment-and-prognosis

Hagin, K. E. (1991). *Faith study course*. RHEMA Bible Church, aka Kenneth Hagin Ministries. Kenneth Hagin Ministries Inc. Tulsa, OK

Healthline (2018). *8 ways Amyloidosis affects the body.* https://www.healthline.com/ health/amyloidosis/how-amyloidosis-affects-the-body#1

Mayo Clinic. *Amyloidosis-Overview,* (1998-2020). Mayo Clinic. https://www.mayoclinic.org/ diseases-conditions/amyloidosis/symptoms-causes/syc-20353178

Medical News Today (2004-2020*). Rare diseases more common than we think.* https://www.medicalnewstoday.com/articles/326879

National Disorders for Rare Disorders (2020). *What is a rare disease?* https://www.rarediseaseday.org/article/what-is-a-rare-disease

National Amyloidosis Centre (2020). *Introduction to Amyloidosis.* National Amyloidosis Centre. https://www.amyloidosis.org.uk/ essentials/introduction-to-amyloidosis/

Price, B. R. (1997). *Through the fire & through the water: My triumph over Cancer.* Faith One Publishing, Los Angeles, CA

Price, F. K. C. (2001). *How faith works.* Faith One Publishing. Los Angeles, CA

Schlosser, B. J., Prigyl, M., & Mirowki, G. W., (2011). *Oral manifestations of hematologic and nutritional diseases.* Otolarynogol Clin N Am. Oto.theclinics.com

Schwartz, D. J. (1959). *The magic of thinking big.* Prentice-Hall Inc., New York, NY

Trimm, C. (2007). *Commanding Your Morning.* Charisma House. Lake Mary, FL

Warren, R. (2002). *The Purpose Driven Live.* Zondervan. Grand Rapids, MN

CONTACTS

If you'd like to contact me for bulk purchases, have questions, or would like to discuss with me speaking engagements
please contact me at:
Email:
<u>yousayihavewhat@gmail.com</u>
Social Media
FB @ **drdeztranscends**

www.ingramcontent.com/pod-product-compliance
Lightning Source LLC
Chambersburg PA
CBHW022103160426
43198CB00008B/337